Robin Ellis is best known as havi... BBC classic serial, *Poldark*, playin... regarded as one of the most popu... produced, beloved in more than forty countries. Robin returned to television to play a cameo in the new twenty-first-century adaptation of the series, produced by Mammoth Screen on behalf of the BBC and PBS/Masterpiece – enchanting a new generation of TV viewers.

Other TV and film appearances have included roles in *Fawlty Towers*, *Elizabeth R*, *Blue Remembered Hills*, *The Good Soldier* and *The Europeans*. He had a long and successful career in British theatre too, including a stint with the Royal Shakespeare Company.

In 1999, Robin was diagnosed with Type 2 diabetes. Although he had no symptoms, he took the diagnosis seriously as his mother had suffered with Type 1 diabetes. In the same year, he and his wife, Meredith, moved to southwest France, where he has become known locally as *l'Anglais who cooks*! By changing the way he ate and taking more exercise, Robin was able to control his blood sugar sufficiently to avoid taking medication for six years. Inspired by a lifelong passion for cooking, he wrote his first cookbook, *Delicious Dishes for Diabetics: A Mediterranean Way of Eating,* in 2011. His second cookbook, *Healthy Eating for Life: Over 100 Simple and Tasty Recipes* (2014), is aimed at everyone wanting to eat more healthily without sacrificing good taste. His third cookbook, *Mediterranean Cooking for Diabetics* (2016), is complemented by over two hundred colour photographs. His updated memoir, *Making Poldark* (2015), also touches upon the positive effect his diagnosis ultimately had on his lifestyle.

Robin blogs regularly on food, cooking and life in rural France at https://robin-ellis.net. He also leads popular healthy cooking workshops in Lautrec, France, famous for its pink garlic festival.

In this wonderful recipe collection Robin shares his favourite vegetarian dishes so that other Type 2 diabetics and their families can enjoy the benefits of a healthy Mediterranean style of cooking.

There's an old Basque saying:

'To know how to eat is to know enough.'

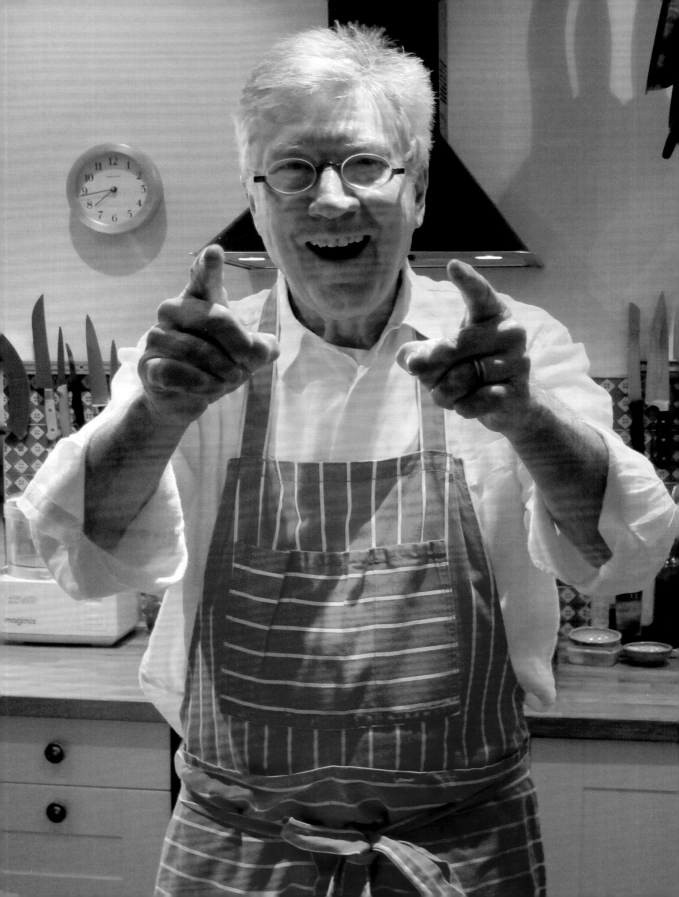

Robin Ellis's
Mediterranean
Vegetarian Cooking

ROBIN ELLIS

Photography by Meredith Wheeler

ROBINSON

ROBINSON

First published in Great Britain
in 2020 by Robinson

10 9 8 7 6 5 4 3 2 1

A CIP catalogue record for this book
is available from the British Library.

ISBN: 978-1-47214-314-3

Designed by Thextension
Typeset in Essay Text
Printed and bound in China
by C&C Offset Printing Co., Ltd.

Papers used by Robinson are from
well-managed forests and other
responsible sources.

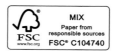

Robinson
An imprint of
Little, Brown Book Group
Carmelite House
50 Victoria Embankment
London EC4Y 0DZ

An Hachette UK Company
www.hachette.co.uk

www.littlebrown.co.uk

HOW TO BOOKS are published by
Robinson, an imprint of Little,
Brown Book Group. We welcome
proposals from authors who have
first-hand experience of their
subjects. Please set out the aims of
your book, its target market and its
suggested contents in an email to
howto@littlebrown.co.uk.

prepared by Robin – with the commitment, love and detail of a great actor preparing for a classical role. Once tasted, never forgotten!'

Lindsay Duncan *actress*
'Robin is the perfect cook to have as a friend. He loves food, cooks superbly and likes nothing more than sharing his food with as many people as he can get round a table. Generosity is at the heart of good cooking and Robin cooks to give pleasure. It always works.'

Romaine Heart *retired cinema-owner (Screen on the Green/the Hill/ Baker Street)*
'Robin's cooking did what five different medications failed to do: bring down my high blood pressure. I suffered a stroke and no medication brought my blood pressure below 177/70. After staying only one week with Robin and eating his delicious meals, it came down to 120/59. How home, my challenge is to reproduce his way of eating. With the help of this cookbook, I am sure I can.'

Michael Pennington *actor and author*
'Robin Ellis has the gift of writing recipes that you can taste as you read them. As if his acting weren't enough, he's now given us a marvellous book – without any pretension or carry-on, just deep affection and knowledge. Absolutely delicious.'

Imelda Staunton *actress*
'How can food this good be this good for you!'

Timberlake Wertenbaker *playwright (Our Country's Good)*
'I've used Robin's recipes again and again. They're elegant, delicious, imaginative and easy to use.
'The Basques are great cooks and giving a dinner in the Basque Country is scary. One also eats very late, so no one wants anything too heavy. I always use one of Robin's recipes and end up with nothing but compliments and a demand for the recipe.

'"An Englishwoman who can cook tuna!" someone said to me in complete astonishment. Of course, the recipes was Robin's.'

contents

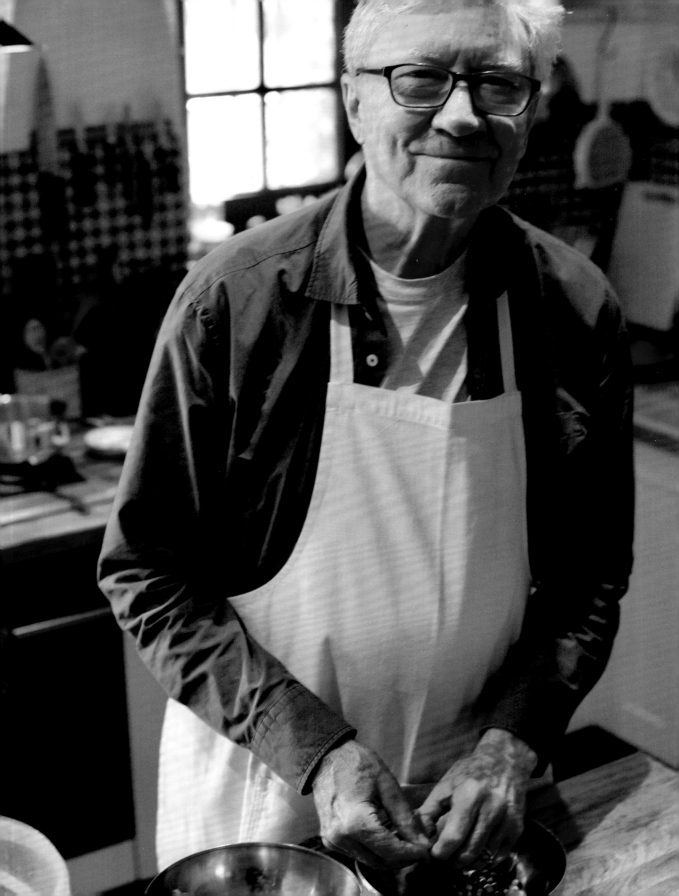

appreciations

This is my fourth book of recipes and I am very lucky to be able to say that. I'm indebted to a number of people for my good fortune. Judith Mitchell was my editor and sympathetic guide for the first two books before she retired from publishing to pursue her passion for genealogy – in which realm we have happily renewed our relationship.

Duncan Proudfoot at Little, Brown has been greatly supportive and encouraging throughout the ten years I've been walking down this new path. Always positive but realistic with his prompt replies to emails, I look forward to every meeting we schedule. I'm indebted once again to Amanda Keats, whose keen eye and gentle prompting keep me in bounds.

I've made a new acquaintance with this book – Tom Asker of Little, Brown – and the experience has been a delight.

He took over the reins from Nikki Read and Giles Lewis, who produced my third book, *Mediterranean Cooking for Diabetics*. They got me to the starting line with this book before retiring, and I thank them both for sticking with it in these difficult times for publishing.

My wife, Meredith Wheeler, took all the terrific photos for that book to much acclaim and she has done so again for this book. It's a task. Thank you, Meredith – your photos add a different sort of spice to the dishes.

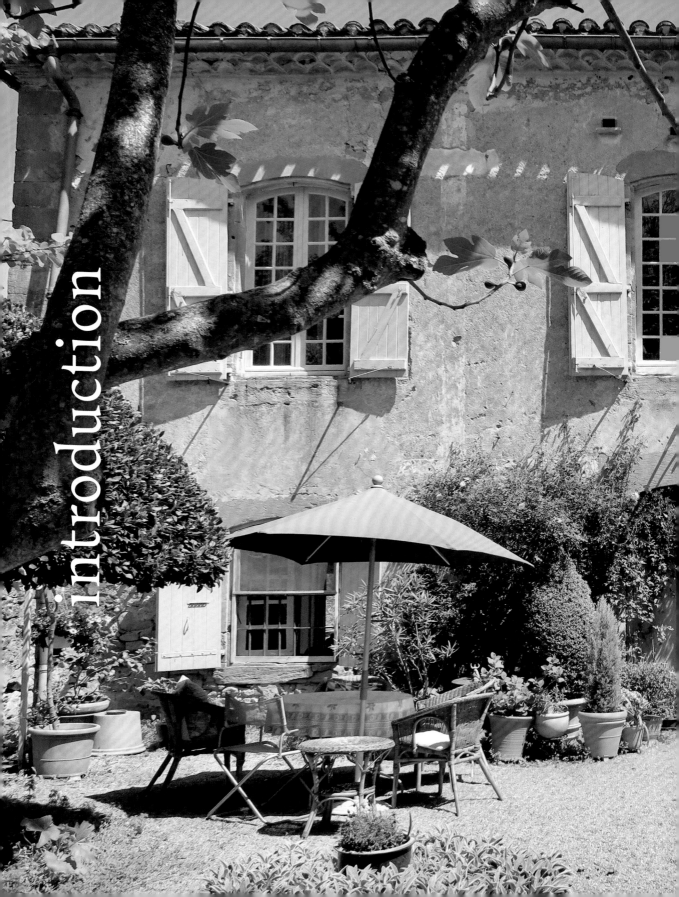

introduction

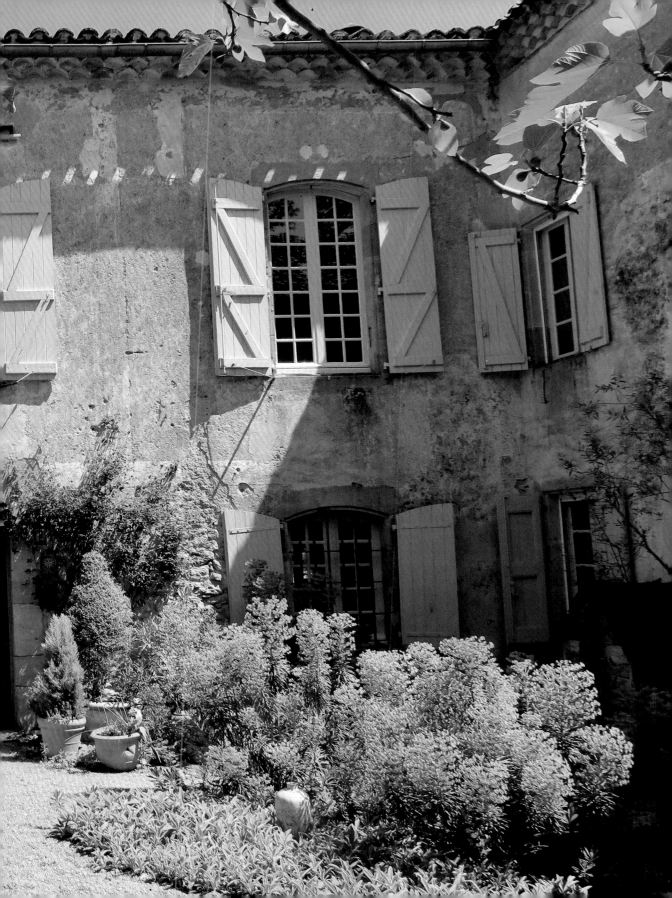

I am not a fully paid-up vegetarian, but I have enjoyed compiling this book, not least because it has meant that we, Meredith and I, have experienced, on a daily basis, the vegetarian way of eating.

Before I set out to write the book, we increasingly found ourselves preferring something vegetarian for supper. We haven't eaten beef for more than 20 years. On the rare occasions that I was buying lamb chops for lunch, I would feel a subtle resistance to cooking them! So the prospect of changing to a mainly vegetarian way of eating for a period was far from a gloomy one and, in any case, I already had a substantial repertoire of veggie recipes tried and tested, to be lined up for possible inclusion.

Whether for ethical or health reasons, vegetarian and vegan ways of eating are in the zeitgeist. Scientists tell us that eating less meat is good for our health and for the planet. This book, however, will not be banging a drum or thumping a tub. I am no missionary. Rather, like Fagin in the song from Lionel Bart's musical *Oliver!*, I am a reviewer of the situation. This book is my way to share the outcomes of my review and to let readers decide.

My first three books are based on the Mediterranean instincts for how to cook and eat. And all three take into account the fact that I am diagnosed with Type 2 diabetes and have to watch what I eat. This book is no different.

The fundamentals of Mediterranean cuisine – olive oil, garlic, pulses, nuts, fruit and vegetables – offer huge scope for a vegetarian cookbook. Look at a map of the region and what hits you is the variety of cultures that edge the Mediterranean Sea, each having its different traditions and methods of cooking. So, in effect, there are many Mediterranean ways of eating, but a shared climate and geography means that each of those traditions uses the same basic ingredients.

In my view, diets are problematic because, by definition, they are restrictive. 'Cut it out!', they cry; 'Give it up!' – they start with a negative. The Med way to eat does not wag a finger. It encourages. The result is that the way we eat can become habitual, an everyday thing, and with any luck something we are *reluctant* rather than *relieved* to give up. This book is about *a way of eating*; it is definitely not about a diet.

'We've lost the seasons'

Wise words from my Geordie driver as he drove us to the studio in Bristol to film my last scene in the last episode of the last series of *Poldark*. Winston Graham's epic family saga has been very good to me over forty years, ever since we made the first series in 1975. So getting togged up for the last time was a moment of some poignancy.

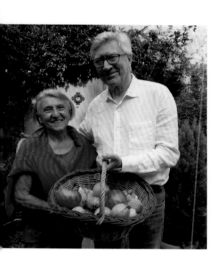

Steve, our driver, is right: things are shifting; these days global warming is starting to play havoc with the seasons. I spotted a headline not long ago that read, 'Italy sees 57% drop in olive harvest as a result of climate change'. There is no doubt that the seasons are no longer so well defined and the weather they bring, dependable.

Garlic gath'rers pass,
Leaving the scent in the air;
It's that time again –

When I started to write this cookbook at the beginning of July, the new garlic was being lifted – normally a sure sign that summer was kicking in. But June had not exactly been 'bustin' out all over' and the garlic quality – as last year – was threatened.

Alice Frezouls, our neighbour and source of country wisdom, had just delivered a truss of the new garlic. Last year's crop was badly affected by blight. Eighty per cent of the harvest was lost, we were told.

'Any better than last year, Alice?'
'Pas vraiment – trop de pluie.' *Rain is the culprit this year.*

I've learned, living here for twenty years, a little understanding of the way farmers cope and to respect their fortitude and fatalism. *C'est comme ça* is an expression you hear often in la France profonde – usually accompanied with the familiar gallic shrug. *That's how it is! What can we expect?* An acceptance that nothing is for certain in the countryside in an increasingly precarious environment.

Suddenly summer
Bursts – in the fields, on the stands;
Yellow, red, golden

What has been very encouraging, though, in recent years is the number of young producers appearing with their produce – mostly organically grown vegetables – at the markets I love to go to each week. It is seasonal stuff and wonderful to have on hand – especially while I've been preoccupied with compiling a vegetarian cookbook.

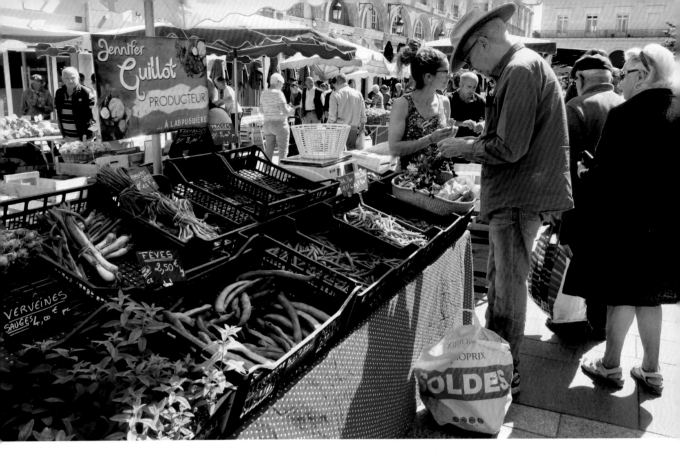

Following the seasons, letting them lead the way in what you choose to cook, for me, is the key to a happy kitchen – that and knowing where your saucepan lids are.

Tomatoes, courgettes,
Aubergines; all in a row—
Ratatouille patch.

Of course, everything is available at any time in the supermarkets, but it would feel strange to me now to be cooking aubergines in December. So it makes sense to divide this book into four sections: Spring, Summer, Autumn and Winter.

There is, of course, no set date when tomatoes disappear from the stalls or on which it is forbidden to eat broccoli. Seasons may be marked on a calendar but not always so accurately in the natural world. Seasonality is approximate; availability, certainly of organic crops, not guaranteed – even more so now with climate change kicking in.

Mediterranean Vegetarian Cooking

Mediterranean vegetarian cooking for Type 2 diabetes

The question those diagnosed with diabetes will want answered is this: is it safe for someone with diabetes to follow a vegetarian way of eating?

And the answer from diabetes charity organisations in the UK and USA is an emphatic YES!

Diabetes UK says:

'Vegetarian diets have been shown to be beneficial for people with Type 2 diabetes, where weight loss is often the most effective way to manage the condition ... with the increased risk of cardiovascular disease in people with diabetes, keeping your weight under control and reducing blood pressure and blood cholesterol are all essential, and plant-based foods can help with these.[*]'

They are, however, keen to emphasise the importance of a balanced diet – which is true for everyone regardless of whether or not they are diabetic. The key for diabetics is to ensure you get enough protein and healthy fat and choose high-fibre carbohydrates and the Mediterranean way of eating hits the mark.

In terms of carbohydrates, a useful guide are the GI index and the GL index.

[*]
www.diabetes.org.uk/guide-to-diabetes/enjoy-food/eating-with-diabetes/vegetarian-diets

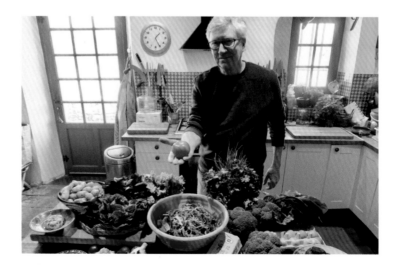

The Glycaemic Index (GI) ranks carbohydrates on a scale of 1 to 100, according to their impact on our blood-glucose levels after eating them. The Glycaemic Load (GL) is a measure of the impact of the glucose in a single *portion* of food.

The GI Foundation neatly sums it up thus:

'Not all carbohydrate foods are created equal. In fact they behave quite differently in our bodies. The glycemic index – or GI – describes this difference by ranking carbohydrates according to their effect on our blood-glucose levels. Choosing low-GI carbs – the ones that produce only small fluctuations in our blood glucose and insulin levels – is the secret to long-term health, reducing your risk of heart disease and diabetes and is the key to sustainable weight loss.'

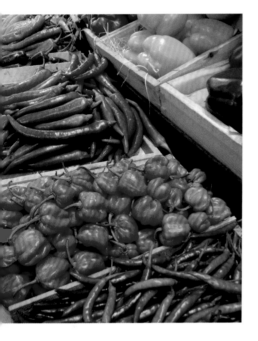

One caveat. If you eat the vegetarian way, you need to take extra care to get enough iron. In my most recent three-monthly test (H1Ac), my doctor noticed I was iron deficient. I told him that Meredith and I were eating vegetarian more than usual because I was in the throes of writing this book. '*Voila!*' he said and prescribed a course of iron tablets.

While the body can store iron, it cannot make it. The Vegetarian Society's recommended daily dose of iron is 8.7mg (this figure increases for women aged 19–50). Iron is found in many green vegetables, such as Brussels sprouts, kale, broccoli and spinach. Growing up I remember loving the cartoon character Popeye the Sailorman, especially the moment when Popeye has to summon up superhuman strength to defeat his arch rival, Bluto, for the affections of Olive Oyl. He swallows large quantities of spinach, transforming his arms into enormously muscled pile drivers! I was so disappointed when my puny arms stayed puny after swallowing gulps of Sainsbury's frozen spinach. I never thought of it at the time, but what a gift to parents trying to get their children to eat more vegetables.

In addition to green vegetables, other food sources of iron are pulses such as lentils, chickpeas and beans; nuts and seeds; and dried fruit.

Protein is vital, too. Pulses, nuts and seeds are good protein sources, as are eggs, cheese and yoghurt. It's important to eat a variety daily.

That's the practical side. It is very important, but for any prescribed or restricted way of eating to be sustainable you have to *enjoy* and *look forward* to mealtimes.

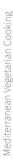

Mediterranean Vegetarian Cooking

In good company: tomatoes and breadcrumbs

The list of well-known vegetarians is long. It includes Mahatma Gandhi, Leonardo da Vinci, Leo Tolstoy, Paul McCartney, Voltaire and the phenomenally prolific playwright George Bernard Shaw. GBS became a vegetarian in 1881 at the age of 25.

'Animals are my friends and I don't eat my friends'

In 1923 he began an address to the University of London Vegetarian Society, 'The subject of diet is a very interesting one, but no one understands it.' He advised his audience never to tell their hostess that they were vegetarian. If they did, he said, she would consult with her cook, and on arrival at dinner the poor vegetarian would be confronted with tomatoes and breadcrumbs – 'horrible stuff'.

I once turned up at a dinner party with the ingredients for my supper – a bag of onions – and proceeded to cook them in my hostess's kitchen and then eat them at her table. I was on the onion diet and my hostess should have shown me the door. Onions are full of goodness, but there are limits.

I have acted in two of George Bernard Shaw's plays, *Widowers' Houses* and *Arms and the Man*. If I'd met Bernard Shaw, I'd have thanked him for writing those and reassured him that with the right tomatoes and a good recipe, tomatoes and breadcrumbs make a very acceptable supper.

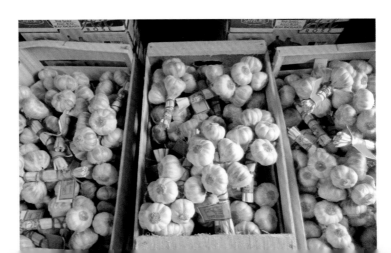

stuffed tomatoes

or *Toms with breadcrumbs – a not-so-bad alternative dinner party dish, served with a green salad!*

Lovely summer-sun-ripened tomatoes are best for this, but we had them for a post-Christmas dinner the other day and the tasty, crisp topping mixed in nicely with the bland tomato flesh.

SERVES 4

4 larger-than-average tomatoes

2 tbsp olive oil, plus extra for brushing and drizzling

2 tbsp wholegrain breadcrumbs

1 garlic clove, finely chopped

2 tbsp finely chopped flat-leaf parsley,

2 tbsp grated Parmesan

salt and freshly ground black pepper

1 Preheat the oven to 180°C/350°F.

2 Carefully slice off the tops of the tomatoes, leaving about three-quarters of each tomato to be stuffed. Reserve the tops. Line a baking tray with foil and brush with oil. Place the main sections of the tomatoes on the tray.

3 Make the stuffing. Put the breadcrumbs in a small bowl and add the garlic, parsley and 2 tablespoons of olive oil. Season with salt and pepper and mix everything together thoroughly. Taste and adjust the seasoning if necessary.

4 Using a teaspoon, scoop out a little of the tomato flesh to make room for some stuffing.

5 Then, carefully pile some stuffing into each tomato, pressing down gently. Place a teaspoon of Parmesan on top of each stuffed tomato and drizzle with a little olive oil.

6 Turn over the sliced tops of the tomatoes so that they are cut-side upwards and place them beside the stuffed tomatoes on the tray. Repeat for the remaining stuffing and Parmesan.

7 Cook in the upper part of the oven for 1 hour, checking for doneness after 40 minutes.

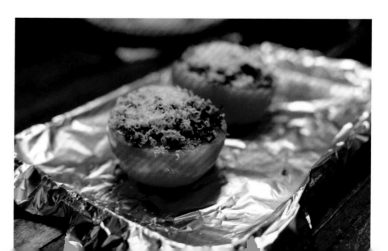

I was eight years old when GBS died in November 1950, aged an impressive 94, making him a great role model for the vegetarian way of eating! I remember hearing the announcement of his death on the radio and seeing his white-bearded image on the front page of our newspaper. He was cremated just down the road from where we were living.

Nothing about his writing or his way of eating registered with me then, but maybe it did with my mother. We ate plenty of home-grown vegetables (Dad's department) and they were not overcooked (Ma's department). This is perhaps the reason that I have never lived in fear and loathing of vegetables as many people do today.

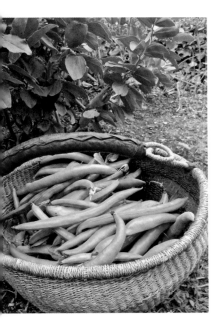

Eureka moment!

Our friend and neighbour, Joan Scott, who grows stupendous vegetables and shares them generously, recently gave me a copy of Deborah Madison's magnificent tome *Vegetarian Cooking for Everyone*. A short sentence in the introduction caught my eye: 'The advantage of using good ingredients is that they allow us to cook simply and eat well.'

Reading that, I made the connection for the first time (it's only taken me 65 years!): Dad's vegetables (I fell in love with his runner beans), Ma's cooking of them and our family custom of eating together around the kitchen table clearly established in me, albeit unconsciously, the joy that comes from such a tradition.

This is not news to our French friends, as playwright Jean Anouilh attests: 'Everything ends this way in France – everything. Weddings, christenings, duels, burials, swindlings, diplomatic affairs – everything is a pretext for a good dinner.'

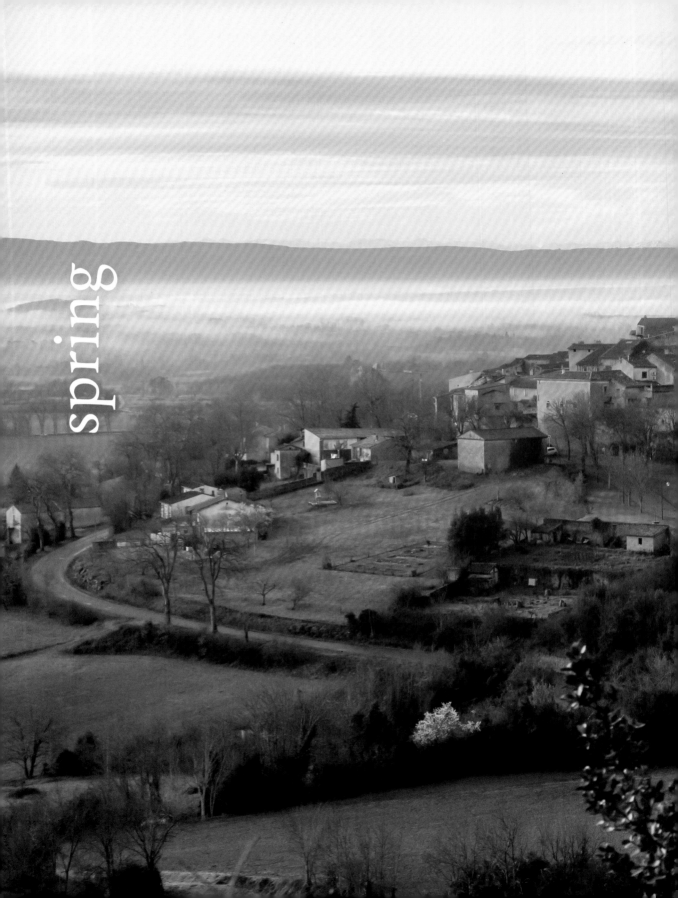

spring

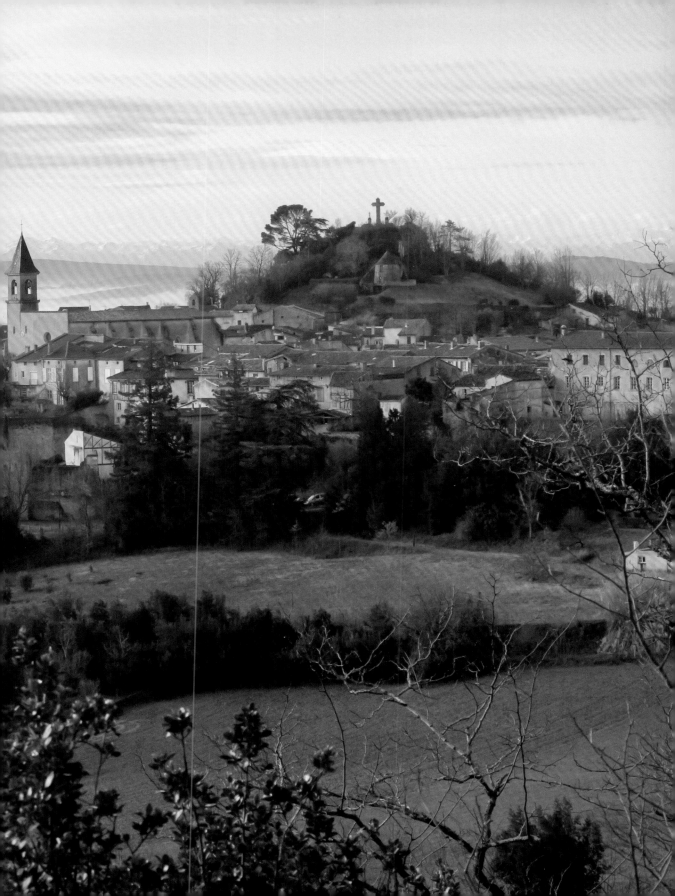

Spring. The word speaks for itself.
Spring to life.
Spring in one's step.
Spring tide.
Spring clean.
Spring fever.

It has the sense of waking up from an enforced period of slumber. There is movement after months of not much movement at all. Nature is moving.

The trees around us are well on their way to blossom and leaf; they are early this year. Bees at work in them, buzzing busily. The birds are on the wing or as the anonymous verse has it:

The spring is sprung, the grass is riz.
I wonder where the boidie is.
They say the boidie's on the wing.
But that's absoid. The wing is on the boid.

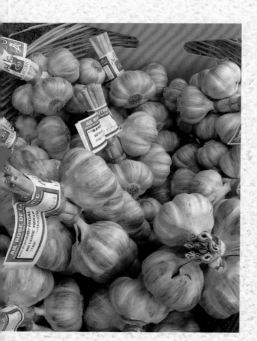

Dad, remembering his wartime visit to New York City in 1944 (en route to Arizona to train to be a fighter pilot), was inspired at this time of the year to dust off his Brooklyn accent and impress us with this piece of joyful nonsense.

Springtime is a time of rebirth, renewal. A hopeful time. The trees around us stagger their re-emergence in a slow firework display that goes on for a month. The oaks are the last and they leave it late as the old, dead leaves are pushed off the branches by the new. We have a number of self-planted trees. Two peaches, a hawthorn, a box elder and, in the courtyard, a fine, upstanding Judas tree that is about to blossom into hot pink. It's a sight!

In table terms not a stellar season.

Spring greens, young spinach and spring onions start popping up on the stalls; but the one main attraction, asparagus, might keep us waiting; it's a star after all.

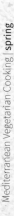

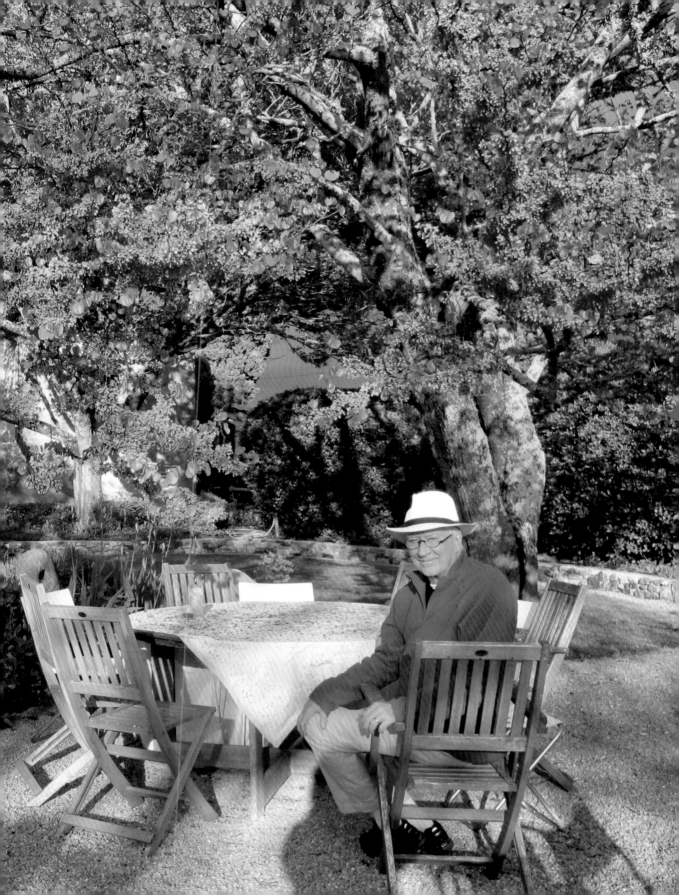

Two welcome spring arrivals combine to brighten the table and lift the spirits. The spinach is there to perk up the dull green of the cooked asparagus.

asparagus soup with spinach

SERVES 4

1 tbsp olive oil

25g/1oz unsalted butter

2 shallots or 1 sweet onion, sliced

1 garlic clove, pulped with a pinch of salt

300g/10oz asparagus, woody ends removed, roughly chopped, a few tips left whole to garnish

800ml/3⅓ cups vegetable stock

30g/1 cup spinach leaves

salt and freshly ground black pepper

1 tsp crème fraîche or yoghurt per bowl

1 Put the oil and butter in a medium saucepan over a low heat and add the shallots or onion and garlic. Sweat gently for 5 minutes, until softened but not browned.

2 Add the asparagus and cook for 2–3 minutes to soften a little. Add the stock and bring to the boil. Reduce the heat to a simmer and leave to cook for 20 minutes.

3 Add the spinach and let it wilt into the liquid for about 2 minutes. Remove the soup from the heat and leave to cool a little before liquidizing it with a hand-held blender. Season to taste. Finish with a teaspoon of crème fraiche or yoghurt and a couple of asparagus tips in each bowl.

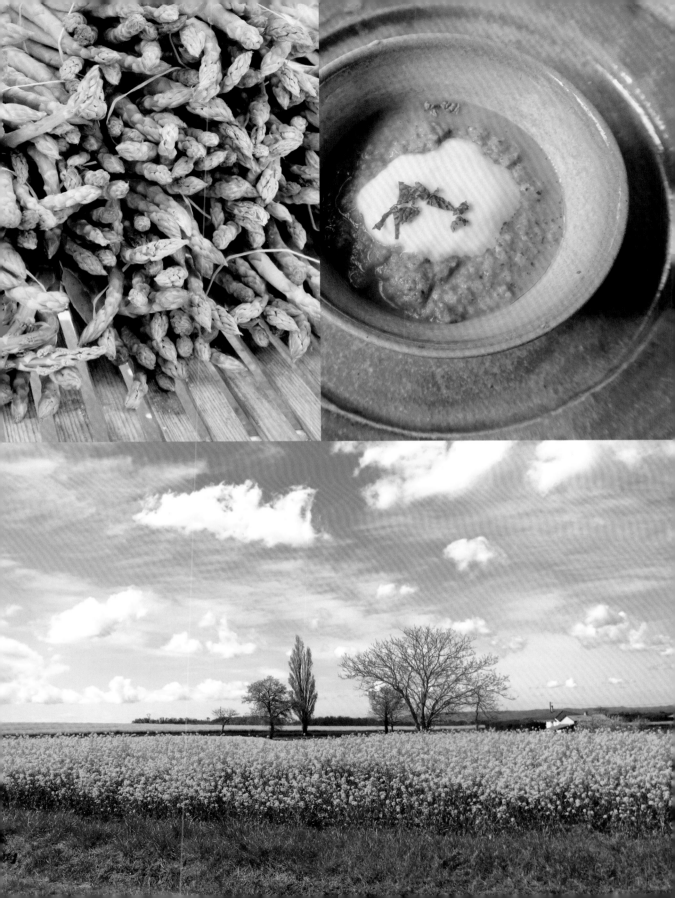

This soup is deliciously fresh and a bit wild looking for the first day of March. You build most winter vegetable soups from the inside out: first by making a soffrito of finely chopped vegetables such as onion, celery and carrot, cooked slowly in olive oil, then adding stock – the taste 'engine room' for a big winter-warming blanket.

But it is 1 March today, so I'm lightening up a little – starting with plain water, adding the ingredients in stages, building the taste and depth gradually, letting the vegetables show off their seasonal colours. The Parmesan and lemon zest topping – sprinkled just before serving – is the hand of spring.

chickpea and vegetable soup

SERVES 5 OR 6

3 tsp salt, plus extra to taste

4 tbsp olive oil

½ onion

2 bay leaves

sprig of rosemary

400g/14oz tin of chickpeas, drained

3 garlic cloves, pulped in a mortar or well-crushed

a small piece of Parmesan rind (optional)

3 carrots, peeled and sliced

3 celery sticks, chopped

400g/14oz tin of plum tomatoes, chopped

½ small cabbage, sliced and roughly chopped

For the Parmesan topping

3 tbsp grated Parmesan

zest of 1 lemon

½ tsp freshly ground black pepper

1 Put 1 litre/4 cups of water in a large pan and bring to the boil. Add the salt, then the oil, onion, bay, rosemary, chickpeas, garlic, and the Parmesan rind, if using. Bring back to the simmer, then cover with a lid.

2 Cook on a low heat for 30 minutes, then add the carrots, celery, tomatoes and cabbage and bring back to the simmer. Cover again and cook for a further 30 minutes, until the vegetables are tender.

3 During the second simmering, prepare the Parmesan topping by mixing together the three ingredients in a bowl.

4 Ladle the cooked soup into bowls and sprinkle the Parmesan topping over just before serving.

Chickpeas – garbanzo in Spanish; pois-chiche in French – are little marvels of protein and carbohydrate with unmatched versatility in the world of pulses. They have been a staple food for millennia. Charlemagne supposedly ate them, although this seems as dubious a claim as 'Elizabeth I slept here'. They make wonderful soup partners as thickening agents – particularly as a substitute for potatoes, which diabetics are better avoiding.

chickpea and fennel soup

SERVES 2 OR 3

400g/14oz tin of chickpeas, liquid reserved

2 small onions, chopped

1 carrot, chopped

1 celery stick, chopped

2 garlic cloves, crushed

4 tbsp olive oil

1 fennel bulb, roughly chopped into large dice

1 thyme sprig and 2 bay leaves, tied together

1 tbsp tomato purée

500ml/2 cups vegetable stock

1 tbsp chopped flat-leaf parsley

salt and freshly ground black pepper

olive oil, to serve

Parmesan, to serve (optional)

1 Put one third of the chickpeas in a blender with some of their liquid and whizz until smooth. Set aside.

2 Sweat the onions, carrot, celery and garlic in the olive oil in a medium saucepan over a low heat for 20 minutes, until softened.

3 Add the blended chickpeas and the remaining whole chickpeas, discarding the rest of the chickpea liquid, to the pan and stir well. Add the fennel, then the tied thyme and bay. Stir in the tomato purée, vegetable stock and parsley.

4 Season well with salt and pepper, bring to the simmer and cook on a low heat for about 25 minutes, until the fennel has softened. Serve in bowls with a swirl of olive oil, and a grating of Parmesan if you wish.

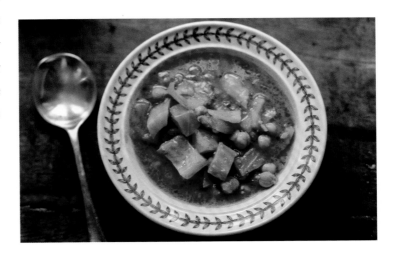

A freezing morning makes this soup a good choice for lunch – just the thought of it warms me up.

I served this smooth wonder to friends who were on a trip from the USA. Mary said it was the best thing she'd tasted in France – I didn't ask how long she'd been here. Pleasingly few ingredients, too.

red lentil soup with lemon

SERVES 4

1 tbsp olive oil

1 onion, diced

4 garlic cloves, crushed

½ tsp ground turmeric

½ tsp ground cumin

300g/1½ cups red lentils

1.25 litres/5¼ cups vegetable stock

juice of 1 lemon

salt, to taste

1 Heat the oil in a large saucepan over a medium–low heat. Add the onion and cook for 5 minutes, until softened. Add the garlic and cook for 2–3 minutes more, until softened but not browned. Stir in the spices and lentils, then add the stock and bring up to the simmer.

2 Cover the pan and cook for 20 minutes, or until the lentils are soft, then stir in the lemon. Check the seasoning, adding salt to taste.

3 Serve with croutons to scatter on top (see opposite).

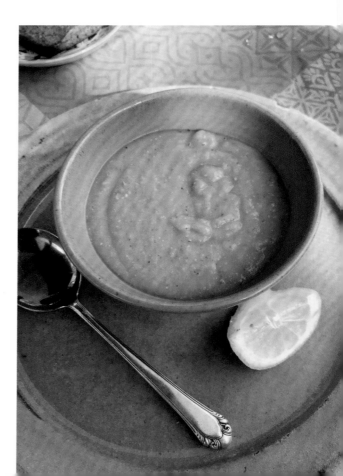

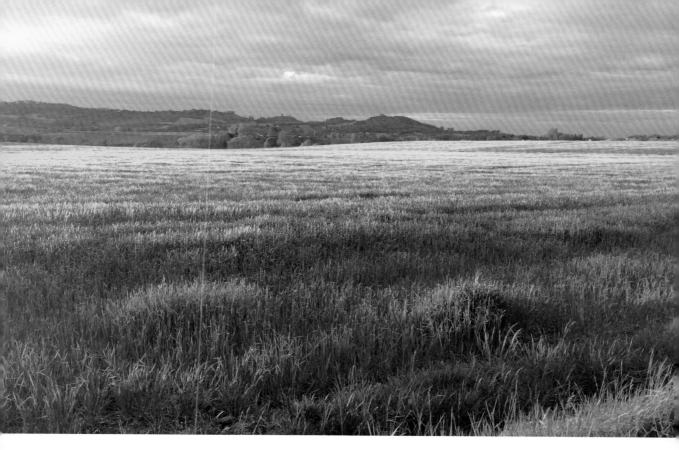

perfect croutons

4 slices of wholemeal or rye
bread per person

1 tbsp olive oil

1 tsp ground cumin or similar spice

salt and freshly ground pepper

1 Pre-heat the oven to 180°C/350°F.

2 Cut the bread into small squares and put them in a mixing bowl. Add the olive oil and mix well to coat. Sprinkle with the cumin, season with salt and pepper and turn to coat.

3 Spread the bread evenly over an oven tray and bake in the top of the oven for 15 minutes, or until the croutons are nicely crisp.

A delicious accompaniment to any
soup, these are so easy to make.

'Caulis', with their big, open faces, urge you to take them home. Meredith grew up thinking that cauliflower was the biggest dud vegetable of all. Fortunately, she has had a conversion!

Like its close relatives, broccoli, Brussels sprouts and cabbage, cauliflower is good for us. One serving contains 77 per cent of the recommended daily intake of vitamin C. It's also a good source of vitamin K, protein, thiamin, riboflavin, niacin, magnesium, phosphorus, fibre, vitamin B6, folate, pantothenic acid, potassium and manganese. So there! We eat it because we like it!

cauliflower and leek soup

SERVES 4

30g/1 oz unsalted butter

3 tbsp olive oil

3 leeks, sliced thinly

1 cauliflower, separated into medium-sized florets

2 bay leaves

1 litre/4 cups vegetable stock

2 tsp salt

freshly ground black pepper

1 Gently melt the butter with the oil in a large saucepan. Add the leeks, cover the pan, and sweat them gently for about 7 minutes or until soft. Add the cauliflower and bay leaves and mix well.

2 Increase the heat a little, pour in the stock and bring to the boil, then lower the heat to a simmer and cook for about 10 minutes until the cauliflower is tender.

3 Add the salt then season with a few good grindings of pepper, to taste.

4 Using a slotted spoon, remove a few small florets from the pan and set aside. Use a hand-held blender and blitz the remainder of the mixture in the pan, until smooth. (Alternatively, transfer the soup to a blender and liquidize until smooth.)

5 Serve with a few florets dropped in each bowl, to garnish.

This recipe is a good example of how it's possible to eat simply, healthily, deliciously and inexpensively.

A tasty variation on my favourite way to cook asparagus, this is best with a thinner variety of this wonderful spring vegetable. It's also quick to make as your guests settle at the table.

roasted asparagus with parmesan

SERVES 3 OR 4

500g/1 lb 2oz thin asparagus

olive oil

salt

2–3 tbsp finely grated Parmesan

1 Preheat the oven to 200°C/ 400°F.

2 Snap off the asparagus ends at the snapping point (where they stop bending) and lay the spears in an even layer on a baking tray. Sprinkle with oil and salt, then roast near the top of the oven for 5 minutes.

3 Remove the tray from the oven. Sprinkle over the Parmesan, then return the tray to the oven for a further 5 minutes. (These times are approximate, depending on the thickness of the spears.)

4 Test for doneness with the tip of a kitchen knife.

5 Finger food really, among friends!

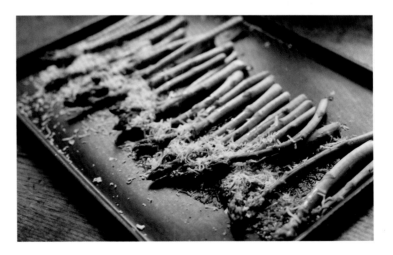

As venerable as prawn cocktail but no less tasty for that, this dish is always a conversation starter – a plus. Undoing the parcel and leaning into the aroma is another plus. It's also simple to assemble and takes just 20 minutes in the oven to cook – a third plus! Use dried herbs if fresh aren't available. You'll need a piece of foil or baking paper roughly 30cm x 30cm/12 x 12in to make the parcel: foil is easier to seal than paper.

champignons en papillotte (mushrooms in a parcel)

SERVES 1

100g/3½oz mushrooms of choice, chopped into bite-sized pieces

½ garlic clove, chopped

a pinch of chopped thyme

a pinch of chopped mint

1 tsp crème fraîche

1 tsp ricotta (optional)

1 tbsp olive oil

salt and freshly ground black pepper

1 Preheat the oven to 200°C/400°F.

2 Lay out your foil or baking paper for the parcel and pile on the mushrooms. Add the garlic, herbs, crème fraîche, ricotta (if using) and olive oil, then season with salt and pepper.

3 Hold the two corners nearest you and fold the foil over the mushroom mixture to meet the two corners farthest away from you. Fold back the edges of the foil on all sides to create an airtight seal. If using baking paper, gather the edges over the mushrooms to form a bag and tie with string. Put the parcel on a shallow oven tray and bake for 20 minutes.

4 Now undo and lean in!

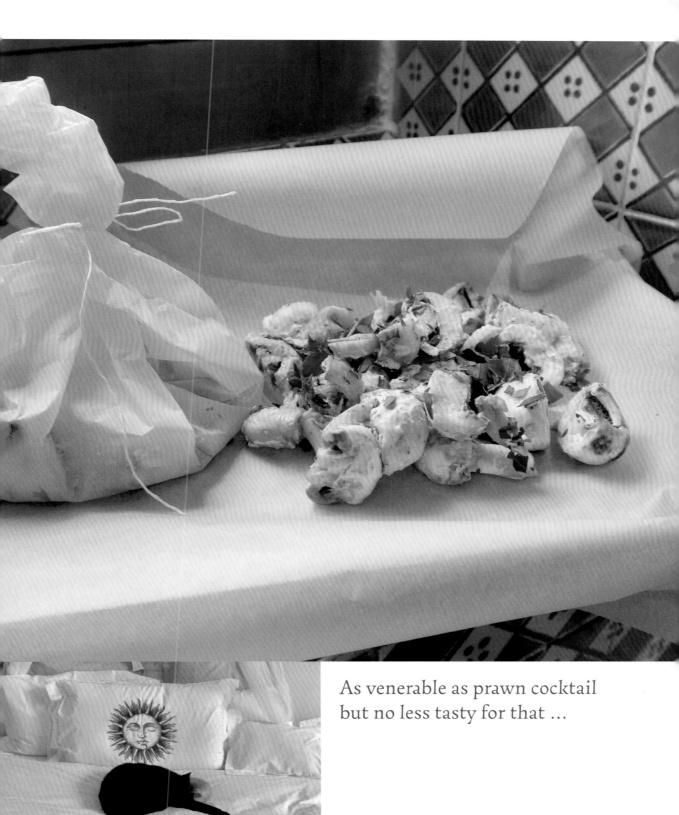

As venerable as prawn cocktail
but no less tasty for that …

Chickpea bread goes by a number of names (and several shapes) – socca, farinata di ceci, foccacia di ceci – depending where you find it. It is street food and I call it chickpea flatbread. There's a recipe for it in my book, Mediterranean Cooking for Diabetics, *but here is a variation.*

I'm going to buy some spring onions in the market tomorrow – well it is spring, after all – grill them as in A Lovely Mess of Spring Onions (see p.36) and spread them over the bread. The sun is forecast, so with any luck we'll eat lunch in the courtyard! Joy!

chickpea flatbread

MAKES 1

580ml/scant 2½ cups sparkling water

230g/2½ cups chickpea flour

1 tsp baking powder

2 tsp salt

2 tbsp olive oil

½ small red onion, finely sliced

1 or more tbsp rosemary needles

freshly ground black pepper

1 Pour the water into a large glass bowl. Sift in the flour and baking powder and stir to mix.

2 Add the salt and olive oil and stir again thoroughly.

3 Cover the bowl and leave the mixture to settle for a couple of hours.

4 When you're ready to bake the 'bread', preheat the oven to 200°C/400°F.

5 Stir in the onion and the rosemary then oil an oven tray and line it with baking parchment. A 29.5cm x 39.5cm tray will result in a thinner 'bread' than a 24cm x 30cm tray and more surface to divide up. I have recently used both and found I prefer the result from the larger tray but Meredith preferred the other; in other words, both are worth trying!

6 Gingerly place the tray in the middle of the oven and bake for 35–40 minutes, until browned. Remove from the oven and ease the loaf out of the tray onto a serving board. Grind some pepper over the top and serve in slices.

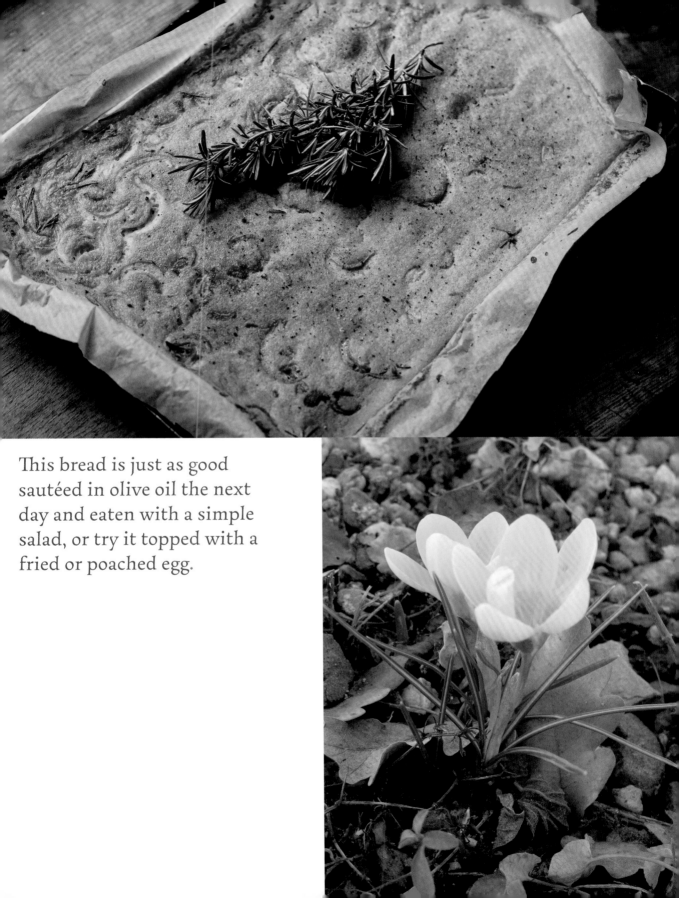

This bread is just as good sautéed in olive oil the next day and eaten with a simple salad, or try it topped with a fried or poached egg.

Not easy to use up a bunch of spring onions in one go, but this recipe makes handy use of the stragglers in the fridge. You may want to add an additional bunch. The size of your griddle/grillpan will determine how many spring onions you can cook at a time.

a lovely mess of spring onions

SERVES 2

a couple of bunches of spring onions

1 tbsp olive oil, plus extra to serve

a pinch of salt, plus extra to season

a squeeze of lemon juice

freshly ground black pepper

1 Heat an iron griddle/grillpan gently until it's hot – shake a hand dipped in water at it and the droplets should sizzle.

2 While the griddle is heating, slice the onions lengthways fairly thinly, taking care not to include a finger in the process. Put them in a bowl, add the olive oil and salt and turn to coat.

3 Spread a layer of onions evenly over the hot griddle so that they all get a chance to char a little. Turn them and rearrange them as they colour up and soften. About 5–7 minutes should do it but it depends on the grill and how many onions you are cooking at one go.

4 Set aside while you cook the next batch.

5 Transfer the cooked onions back to the bowl, sprinkle with lemon juice and a little more oil and season with salt and pepper.

A word of warning: once you start eating spring onions like this, it's hard to stop picking at the pile on the serving plate.

This comes in handy eaten either as a main course – as we did for lunch today – or to accompany a dish of lentils, perhaps. The yoghurt sauce (see p.210) adds a grace note.

cauliflower with olive oil, rosemary and garlic

SERVES 3 OR 4

1 cauliflower, cut into bite-sized pieces

3 tbsp olive oil

4 garlic cloves, pulped in a mortar with a pinch of salt

1 tbsp rosemary needles, finely chopped

1 tsp salt

4 grindings of black pepper

juice of 1 lemon

1 Preheat the oven to 230°C/450°F.

2 Place the cauliflower pieces in a large bowl.

3 In a separate, small bowl mix together the oil, garlic, rosemary, salt and pepper and pour the mixture over the cauliflower. Turn to coat the cauliflower in the garlicky oil.

4 Line a baking tray with foil or baking paper and lightly brush with oil. Tip in the coated cauliflower pieces and spread them out in an even layer. Roast for 20 minutes, until the cauliflower is nicely charred (check after 15 minutes that it is not burning).

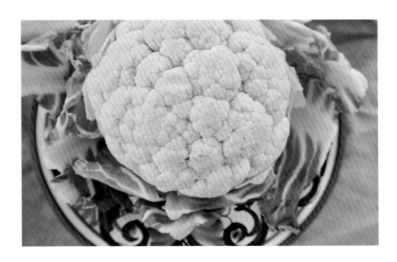

This is tasty and colourful – a refreshing early summer salad that originates from the island of Sicily, apparently. I use a food processor to slice my cucumber to save time.

sicilian cucumber and orange salad

SERVES 4

1 cucumber, peeled and sliced
very thinly in rounds

1 orange, plus 1 tbsp juice

a few radishes, thinly sliced

a handful of torn mint leaves

1 tsp white wine vinegar

1 tsp lemon juice

3 tbsp olive oil

salt and pepper

1 Put the cucumber slices in a colander or sieve and sprinkle some salt over. Leave to drain for 30 minutes, then remove them from the colander and dry them on kitchen paper.

2 Peel the orange down to the flesh (leaving no white pith) – I do this by running a sharp knife around the top of the orange and slicing it off, then turning the orange to slice off the peel and pith in a continuous motion from top to bottom. The knife should be just touching the flesh. Cut the orange into thin rounds.

3 Build the salad prettily – a white dish sets off the colours! – layering the cucumber, orange, radish and mint as you wish.

4 Whisk together the orange juice, vinegar, lemon juice and olive oil. Season to taste, then pour the dressing over the salad. Turn it all over and serve.

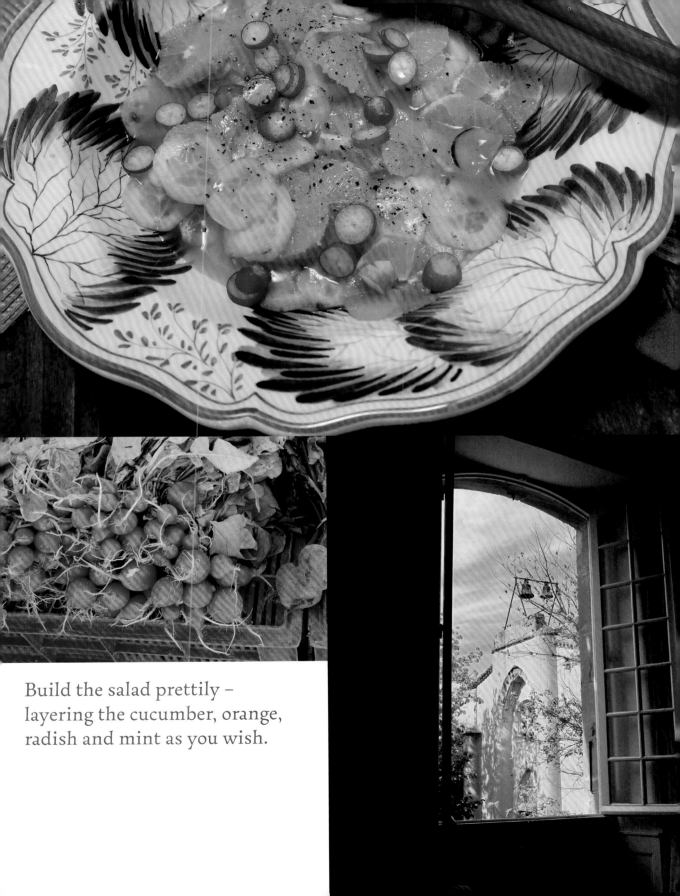

Build the salad prettily –
layering the cucumber, orange,
radish and mint as you wish.

The tahini-based dressing is the thing here. It has the consistency of a runny mayonnaise without the anxiety factor in the mixing of it and it pulls this salad together effortlessly.

herby chickpea salad with tahini dressing

SERVES 4

400g/14oz tin of chickpeas, drained

½ cucumber, roughly chopped

1 red pepper, deseeded and roughly chopped

1 red chilli, deseeded and finely chopped

2 tomatoes, roughly chopped

a handful of mint leaves, finely chopped

a handful of flat-leaf parsley, finely chopped

1 tbsp tahini

2 tbsp red wine vinegar

juice of ½ lemon

4 tbsp olive oil

salt and freshly ground pepper

wholemeal pitta, to serve

1 Put the chickpeas in a bowl and stir in the cucumber, red pepper, chilli, tomatoes and herbs.

2 In a separate bowl, whisk together the tahini, red wine vinegar, lemon juice and olive oil.

3 Pour the dressing over the chickpea mixture, stir, then season with salt and pepper.

4 Serve with wholemeal pitta breads.

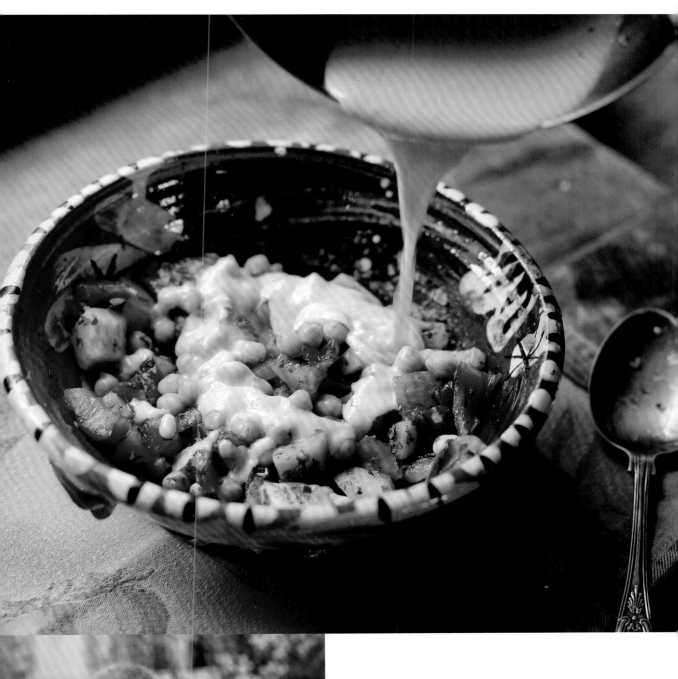

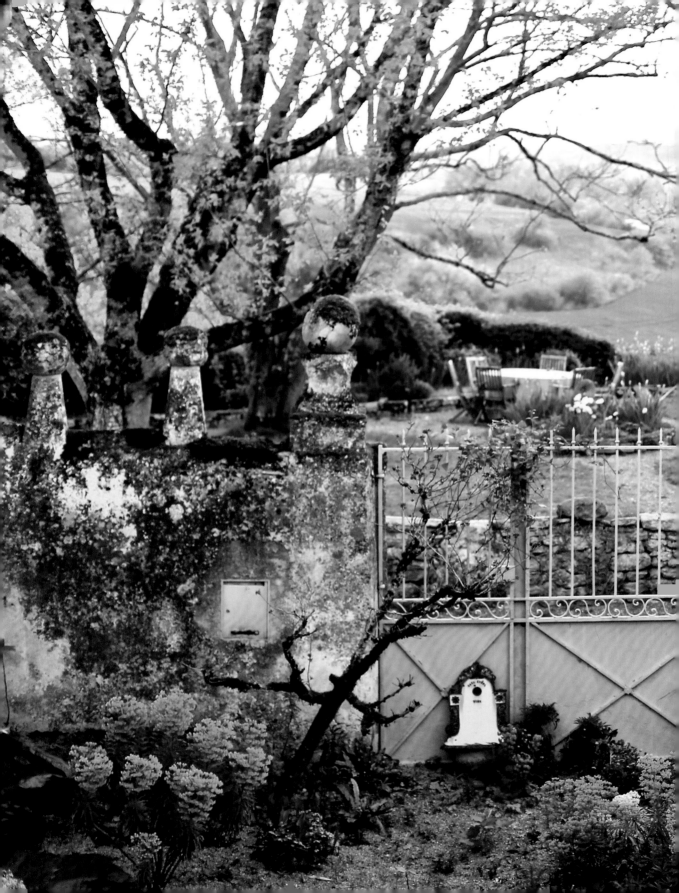

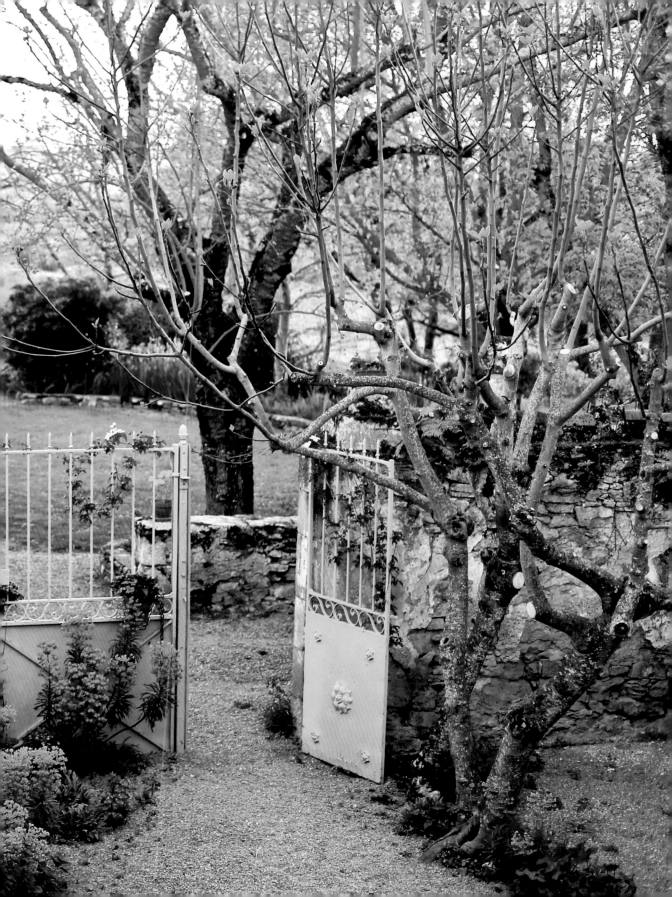

Baby gems are called sucrines *here in France and the name better describes their sweet nature. The stems, though, retain a pleasing bitterness, which nicely contrasts with the unctuous tomato sauce. This is not quite a one-pot meal, but it is served as such.*

white beans in a tomato and black olive sauce with grilled baby gem lettuce

SERVES 4

4 tbsp olive oil

2 large garlic cloves, pulped in a mortar or well-crushed, with a pinch of salt

1½ tsp finely chopped rosemary needles

400g/14oz tin of tomatoes, chopped

400g/14oz tin or jar of white beans, drained

200ml/generous ¾ cup vegetable stock

12 juicy pitted black olives

4 little gem lettuce, quartered

salt and freshly ground black pepper

For the vinaigrette

1 tbsp red wine vinegar

3 tbsp olive oil

1 Heat the oil in a shallow pan and gently fry the garlic and rosemary for about 2 minutes until the garlic begins to colour.

2 Add the tomatoes and cook on a medium–high heat for 5 minutes, stirring often.

3 Stir in the beans and the stock, then cook for about 10 minutes, stirring often, until the sauce has thickened and deepened in flavour.

4 Stir the olives into the thickened sauce, season with salt and pepper to taste and set aside.

5 While the sauce is cooking, heat the griddle over a low heat, and make the vinaigrette by whisking together the vinegar and oil. Use this to brush the lettuce quarters all over, then set them aside.

6 Place the lettuce quarters on the griddle, to soften and char a little. Lay the quarters on the bean mixture in the pan and shake the pan to settle them.

7 Cover the pan and cook for a further 10 minutes to allow the lettuce quarters to integrate thoroughly.

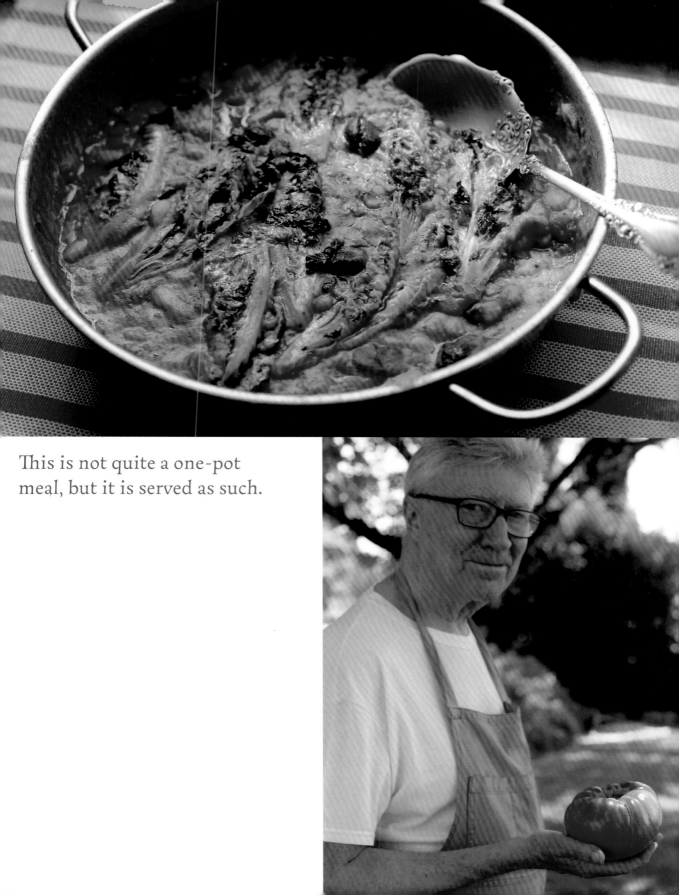

This is not quite a one-pot
meal, but it is served as such.

Little pearls, half the size of their better-known cousins cannellini beans, but cooked the same way, fagioli del purgatorio (literally meaning 'purgatory beans') come from Gradoli, a town about 100 kilometres northwest of Rome. The size of the beans suits this little salad, but you could use any white bean.

One definition of purgatory has it as '... a temporary condition of torment or suffering'. When it comes to eating beans, Meredith would agree and would willingly give them up for longer than Lent! She said today that if she were to take over in the kitchen – something she is capable of doing – she'd cook more or less like I do, except no beans. Meredith grew up near Chicago, the Windy City – perhaps she's had her fill of wind!

little white bean salad

SERVES 2 OR 3

250g/2¼ cups dried fagioli del purgatorio or any white beans, soaked for at least 8 hours in water

1 carrot, halved lengthways

1 celery stick, halved lengthways

1 onion, halved

a sprig of rosemary

1 small red onion, finely chopped

2–3 tbsp chopped flat-leaf parsley

lemon wedges, to serve

For the dressing

4 tbsp olive oil

2 tbsp red wine vinegar

1 garlic clove, pulped in a mortar or well-crushed, with a pinch of salt

salt and freshly ground pepper

1 Preheat the oven to 170°C/340°F.

2 Put the soaked beans, the halved vegetables and rosemary in an ovenproof pan. Pour in enough water to cover by 5cm/2in and bring gently to the boil.

3 Spoon off any white froth that collects on the surface, then cover the pan and place in the middle of the oven. After 30 minutes, check the beans – they should be soft, but not mushy. If they still seem a little crunchy, cook on until they are soft. (The older the beans, the longer they take to cook.)

4 When you are happy that the beans are tender, drain them and discard the onion, celery, carrot and rosemary (they are just there to give flavour during cooking). Tip the beans into a pretty serving bowl.

5 Mix together the dressing ingredients, season with salt and pepper, and pour over the beans while they are still warm. Add the red onion and parsley and carefully turn everything over in the bowl to combine. Serve with lemon wedges for squeezing over.

Note *A fuller definition of purgatory from Merriam-Webster's Collegiate Thesaurus is 'An intermediate state after death for expiatory purification; specifically: a place or state of punishment wherein the souls of those who die in God's grace may make satisfaction for past sins and so become fit for heaven.' Well, I'd be happy to take my punishment – I love beans! Wind or no wind!*

This dish is traditionally served at lunch in Gradoli on Ash Wednesday, which marks the beginning of Lent in the Christian calendar – a time to purge sins by giving up something we enjoy. I remember dreading it as a child in the fifties. No chocolate or sweets for seven weeks – purgatory!

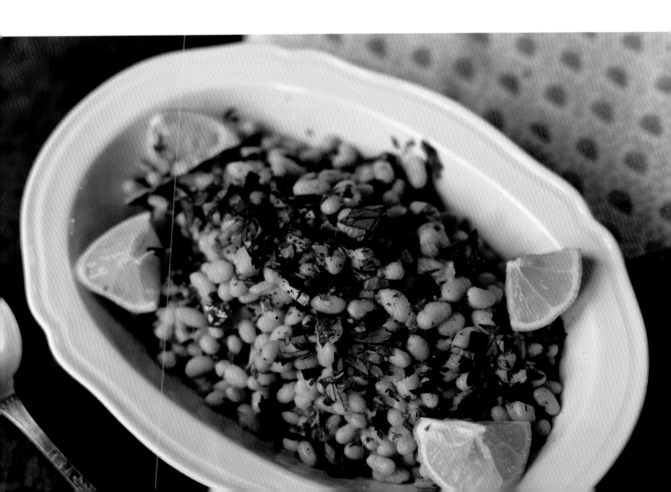

Our friend Hilton McRae, a good cook who loves Italy and knows a thing or two about Italian cooking, gave me this recipe. Fresh borlotti may be hard to find but tinned or jarred are available wherever Italians have settled. They work well for this moreish salad, which he serves with a green salad. 'Dee-licious!' says Hilt. Je suis d'accord!

borlotti bean salad

SERVES 3 OR 4

400g/14oz tin of borlotti beans, drained

1 celery stick, finely chopped

1 carrot, finely chopped

1 red onion, finely chopped

3 tbsp olive oil

1 tbsp lemon juice

4 tbsp Gremolata (see p.210)

salt and freshly ground black pepper

1 Place the beans in a small pan over a low heat, add a couple of tablespoons of water and heat through.

2 Meanwhile, place the vegetables, olive oil and lemon juice in a bowl, then season generously (more than you think) with salt and pepper.

3 Drain the beans, then add the hot beans and the gremolata to the vegetables. Toss to combine and serve the same day (don't refrigerate).

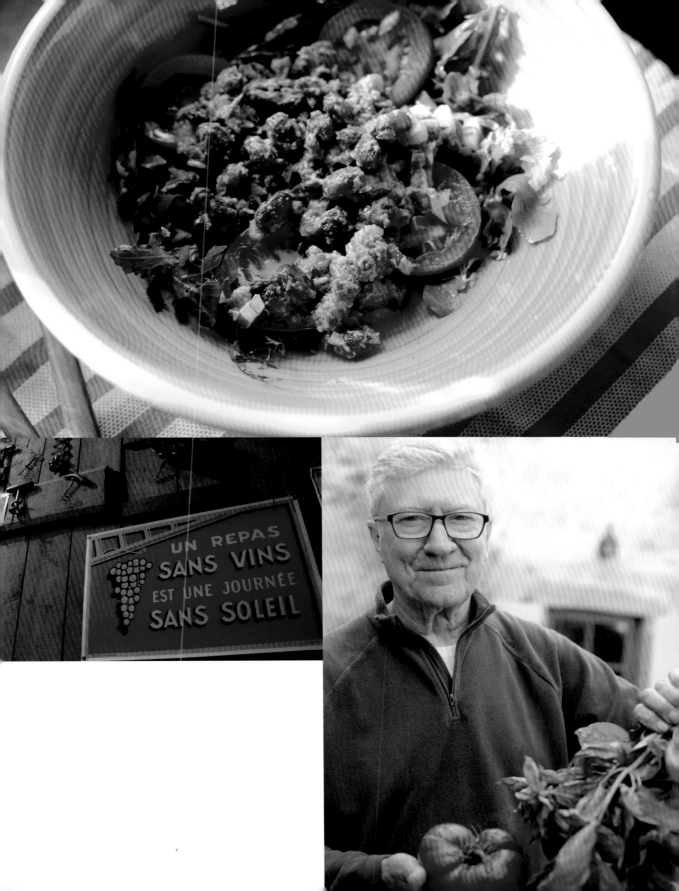

This is my favourite spring dish. The name is beautiful and suggests it has been on the menu for centuries. It is Roman in origin but can be made anywhere the fresh ingredients are available, and as long as there are willing hands to peel and pod.

vignarola

Mediterranean Vegetarian Cooking | spring

SERVES 4

1 lemon, halved, plus extra to serve

3 large artichokes

500g/1lb 2oz broad beans, podded

4 tbsp olive oil, plus extra to serve

3 spring onions, sliced top to toe

150ml/⅔ cup white wine

500g/1lb 2oz peas in their pods, podded

1 small lettuce, shredded

salt and freshly ground black pepper

1 Have a bowl of water to hand, with the juice of half a lemon squeezed into it, to park the artichoke slices and prevent them from discolouring.

2 Prepare the artichokes. One at a time, slice each tail almost to the bulb. Start at the base and, using a small knife if it helps the leverage, pull back and away leaf by leaf, until you have left the pale pinky green interior leaves. Slice off the top half of the artichoke and, working round the base, snap back or scrape off the remaining dark green leaves and discard. The little light green leaves left should be soft enough to eat. Use the point of the knife in a circular movement to scoop out the soft, fluffy choke. Place the artichokes face down on the chopping board and vertically slice them thinly. Drop the slices into the lemony water.

3 Bring a small saucepan of salted water to the boil, then add the beans. Cook for a minute or two and then drain. When the beans are cool enough to handle, squeeze the brilliant green interior bean from its outer casing. Set aside.

4 Heat the oil in a shallow pan. Add the spring onions and a good pinch of salt, then cook gently for about 10 minutes, until softened.

5 Drain the artichoke slices and add them to the pan with the onions, turning to mix. Add 4 tablespoons of the water and the juice of half a lemon to the mixture, along with the wine, then cover the pan.

6 Cook gently for about 20 minutes, until the artichokes are tender. (Cooking time will depend on how thinly you sliced the artichokes.)

7 Add the peas and the lettuce and a little more water if you feel it needs it – there should be a sauce, but take care not to flood the flavour out of it. Cover and cook for 2–3 minutes, then add the broad beans.

8 Turn it all over and for cook a couple more minutes to tenderise the beans.

9 You can serve it hot immediately, or later, tepid, with a swirl of oil and a squeeze of lemon either way.

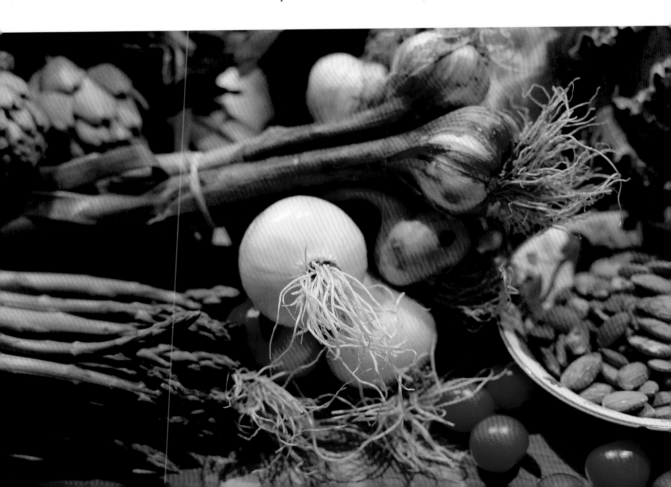

Lovely green asparagus spears were in Realmont market today, at reasonable prices. I bought a kilo of straight ones for Friday dinner with our guests arriving from the USA. I also bought a second batch of less-than-perfect specimens (and less expensive too), asperges tordues, to make this very simple frittata for lunch. This recipe gives you something different to do with a vegetable that has a relatively short-lived season, and provides a use for the cheaper spears with less-than-perfect appearance. I have five eggs left in the pantry and a red onion. Add some cheese and seasoning – and there you have all the ingredients you need! The result is 'high on the ding scale', said Meredith.

asparagus frittata

SERVES 3 OR 4

3 tbsp olive oil

1 red onion, chopped

250g/9oz (trimmed weight) asparagus spears, cut diagonally into small pieces

5 eggs, beaten

50g/2oz Parmesan, grated

salt and freshly ground black pepper

1 Heat 2 tablespoons of olive oil in a medium pan over a medium to low heat. Add the onion and cook for 10–15 minutes, until caramelised.

2 Mix in the asparagus pieces, season with salt and a twist or two of pepper, then cook over a gentle heat for about 10 minutes, until the asparagus begins to soften. I like the pieces to retain a little bite. Remove the pan from the heat and allow the mixture to cool before easing it into the beaten eggs.

3 Fold in the cheese and check the seasoning.

4 Heat the remaining tablespoon of oil in a frying pan with a heatproof handle until hot, and pour in the egg mixture, spreading it out evenly.

5 Immediately turn the heat down to the lowest setting and cook the frittata for 30 minutes, until just a small pool of liquid is left on top.

6 Heat the oven grill to hot then slip the pan under it for about 30 seconds or until the top is firm and golden. Be careful when taking the pan out as it will be very hot (as I was reminded when the pan touched the side of my hand by accident – ouch)!

7 Loosen the frittata round the edges of the pan using a fish slice or spatula and ease it out onto a favourite platter. Serve in wedges with a seasonal salad.

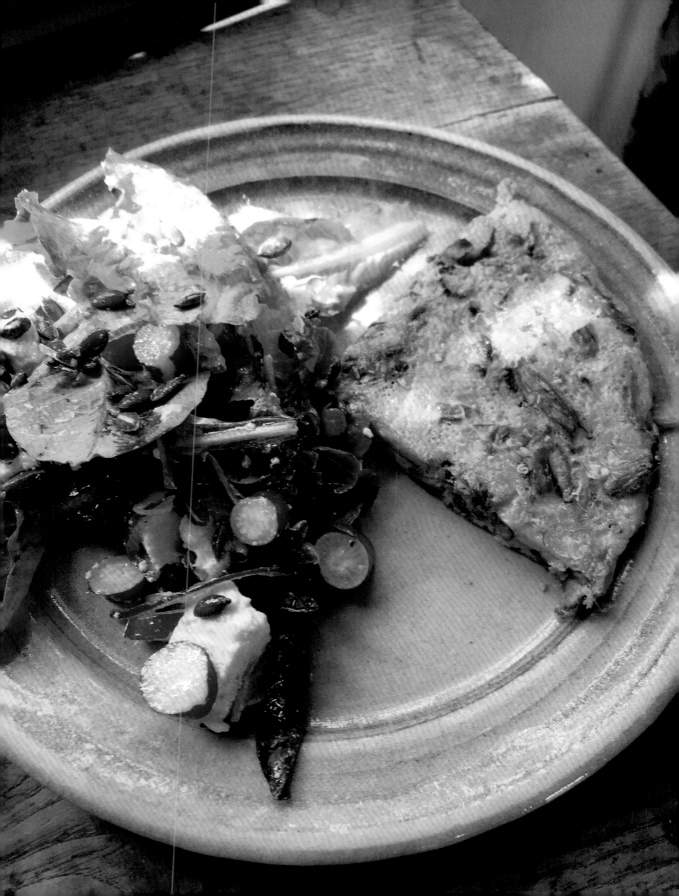

The inspiration for this recipe is in Leaves from Our Tuscan Kitchen, a gem of a book, by Janet Ross and Michael Waterfield. The gratin makes for a satisfying supper – and there is never enough of it!

fennel and tomato gratin

SERVES 4

6 tbsp olive oil

1 large onion, sliced

2 garlic cloves, chopped

4 fennel bulbs, prepared as in recipe on p.55

600g/1lb 5oz ripe tomatoes, skinned and diced

salt and freshly ground black pepper

For the topping

50g/2oz wholemeal or rye breadcrumbs

zest of 1 lemon

1 garlic clove, finely chopped

1 Combine the topping ingredients in a bowl and set aside. Preheat the oven to 200°C/400°F.

2 Heat the oil in a large sauté pan over a medium heat, add the onion and soften for 5 minutes, then add the garlic and cook for 2–3 minutes more. Stir in the fennel, then cover the pan and cook for 10 minutes, until softened and beginning to colour.

3 Mix in the tomatoes and season with salt and pepper. Cover with a lid or piece of foil and cook for 10 minutes, then remove the lid or foil and cook for a further 10 minutes, or until you have a lovely, soft mixture.

4 Spoon the mixture into an ovenproof dish, cover evenly with the topping and bake near the top of the oven for 10 minutes, or until the topping is sizzling.

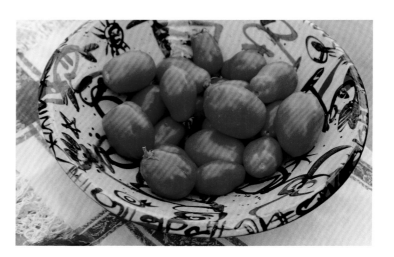

A handy and delicious salad to have in the fridge for lunch with friends on a spring day.

fennel à la grecque

SERVES 3 OR 4

2 fennel bulbs

6 tbsp olive oil

8 coriander seeds

juice of ½ lemon

10 peppercorns

5 juniper berries

1 bay leaf

1 thyme sprig

12 juicy pitted black olives, halved

100g/1¾oz feta cheese or more, cut into small dice

salt and pepper

1 Prepare the fennel bulbs. In turn, place each bulb on its side and slice across 1cm/½in from the bottom. This will release the outer layers and reveal the little white circle at the base. Insert the tip of a sharp knife and work it round the circle to carefully remove – you will have a rounded triangular piece. A satisfying manoeuvre, though take care the knife doesn't slip: your hands and fingers are vulnerable.

2 Slice through the stalks across the top to remove – this may release another outer layer of the bulb.

3 Stand each bulb upright and slice downwards at roughly 1cm/½in intervals. Depending on the size of the bulbs, each should give you about eight slices.

4 Put all the remaining ingredients except the olives and cheese in a large saucepan with 350ml/1½ cups of water and gently bring up to a simmer.

5 Add the fennel slices and cook for about 20 minutes on a low heat, until the fennel is tender.

6 Using a slotted spoon, remove the fennel slices to a serving plate and let the contents of the pan cook for a further 10 minutes to concentrate the flavours. Carefully pour the liquid and its contents over the fennel, then sprinkle over the olive halves and the cubed feta.

Known in Syria as horaa osbao, *this dish has a name that means 'results in burned fingers'. In other words it is so irresistible that you can't wait for it to cool before starting to eat it in the traditional Syrian manner – with your fingers, ouch! These little brown lentils hold their shape. Serve with fried onions (see below).*

syrian brown lentils

SERVES 4

450g/2⅓ cups brown lentils

6 tbsp olive oil

2 onions, finely chopped

4 tbsp chopped flat-leaf parsley or coriander

6 garlic cloves

2 tsp ground cumin

4 tbsp lemon juice

salt and freshly ground black pepper

1 Place the lentils in a large saucepan and cover with water by 2.5cm/1in. Bring to the boil. Cook for about 20 minutes, until tender, but not mushy.

2 Meanwhile, heat the oil in a frying pan over a medium heat and add the onions. Cook for about 5 minutes, until softened. Add the parsley or coriander and the whole garlic cloves and continue cooking for a couple more minutes. Add the cumin and lemon juice, stir to combine, then season with salt and pepper and stir again.

3 When the lentils are cooked, add the contents of the frying pan and stir to combine. Bring the mixture up to a simmer and then reduce the heat to its lowest setting. Cook for 1 hour until the sauce has thickened.

4 This is traditionally served with fried pasta sprinkled on top. Crispy fried onions (see p.152) would be a healthier option for diabetics.

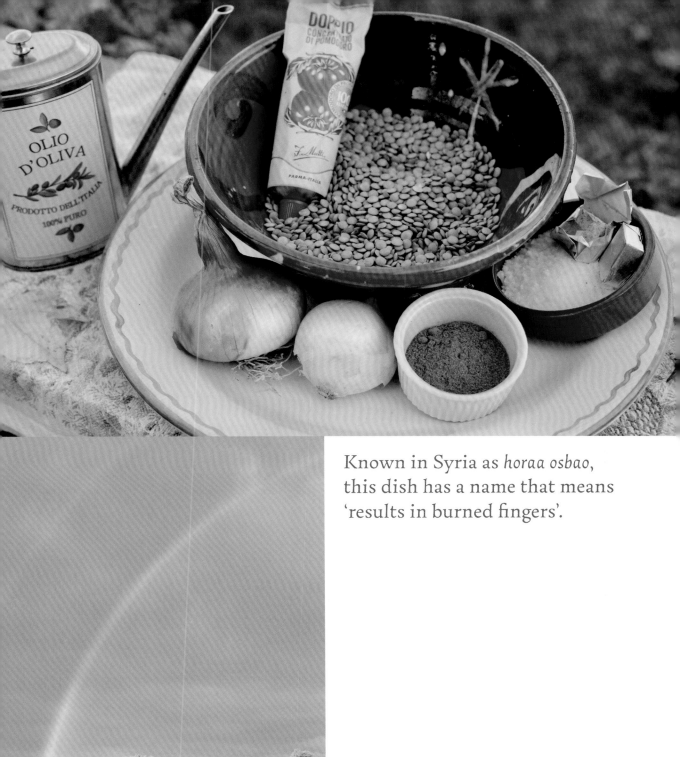

Known in Syria as *horaa osbao*, this dish has a name that means 'results in burned fingers'.

This is soufflé-like and I have wanted to crack a soufflé for years. Never managed it; never dared; never really investigated how to solve the mystery of the fluffy nothingness. This hardly qualifies as a classic soufflé, but it has a delicious fluffy somethingness. Ricotta is made from whey – the liquid left after milk has been curdled and strained to make cheese. It fits the nothingness description.

Cook either in individual ramekins or in a small heatproof dish to serve spooned out in portions.

baked ricotta with thyme and parmesan

SERVES 4

450g/1lb ricotta

2 eggs, beaten

small pinch of *piment d'espelette* or cayenne pepper

1 tsp finely chopped thyme leaves, or a pinch of dried thyme

50g/2oz Parmesan, grated

olive oil, for brushing

salt and freshly ground black pepper

1   Preheat the oven to 200°C/400°F.

2   Empty the ricotta into a bowl and gently mix in the eggs and *piment d'espelette* or cayenne pepper and thyme. Carefully turn in the Parmesan, then season with salt and pepper.

3   Brush the ramekins or baking dish with a little olive oil and fill evenly with the mixture, then place on a shallow oven tray. Cook in the upper part of the oven for about 30 minutes, until the mixture shows a pleasing browning on top. Serve immediately.

4   To contradict King Lear, 'Something has come of nothing.'

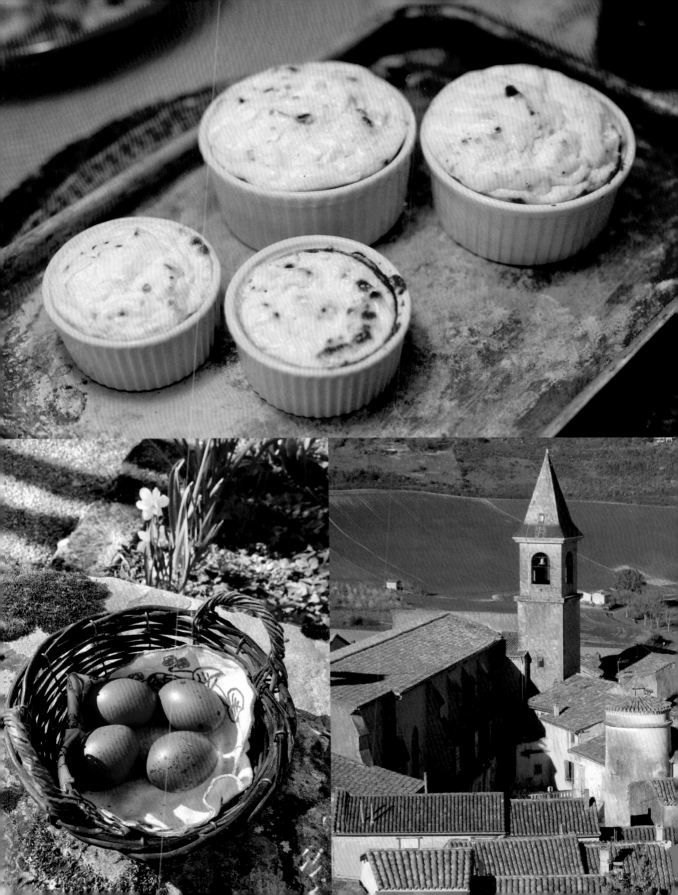

The flavour is pure cauliflower, which I love. The egg(s) on top are optional, but add to the interest. Although, as Meredith said the other day, we seem to be adding an egg to everything.

filigreed roasted cauliflower

SERVES 2–3

1 large cauliflower, leaves removed

olive oil, for brushing

grated Parmesan, to sprinkle

poached or fried egg per person, to serve (optional)

For the dressing

3 tbsp olive oil

1 tbsp red wine vinegar

salt and pepper

1 Heat the oven to 200°C/400°F.

2 Rest the base of the cauliflower on a chopping board, making sure it's secure and won't wobble. Cut top to toe: using a large knife, carefully cut down through the head in roughly 2.5cm/1in-wide slices. It is fascinating to see the thick filigree of this beautiful vegetable in cross-section.

3 Cover a large shallow baking tray with foil and brush with oil. Arrange the cauliflower slices on the tray. (You could tidy the pieces with a sharp knife, but don't cut through the little connecting stems – or your fingers!)

4 Combine the dressing ingredients in a bowl. Generously brush each slice with the dressing and season with salt and pepper.

5 Slip the tray in the top of the oven for about 30 minutes, then turn over the slices, easing them gently off the foil. Top with a generous sprinkling of grated Parmesan and place the tray back in the oven for about another 15 minutes to allow the cheese to melt and brown a little.

6 Serve each portion with a poached or fried egg (optional) and green salad.

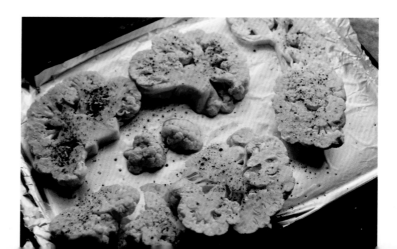

The classic Roman pasta dish of garlic, olive oil and hot red pepper. It is spicy, garlicky and also simple – ready in almost a trice. How hot and how garlicky you make this comes down to personal taste and the experience of eating it.

spaghettini aglio, olio e peperoncino

SERVES 1

100g/3½oz spaghettini

2 tbsp olive oil

2 garlic cloves, pulped in a mortar

2 small dried chillies, chopped small

salt and pepper

chopped parsley, to serve (optional)

1 Cook the pasta in plenty of well-salted boiling water until quite al dente. (How al dente the pasta, like the other choices, is up to you – I couldn't possibly comment, except to whisper that in Italy to overcook pasta is a chargeable offence…)

2 While the pasta cooks, heat the oil in a sauté pan with high sides. Add the garlic and gently fry until it begins to colour. Add the chillies and the drained al dente pasta.

3 Cook for a couple more minutes, turning everything over in the pan to coat the spaghettini with the spicy sauce. Season with salt and pepper to taste and scatter with parsley if you wish.

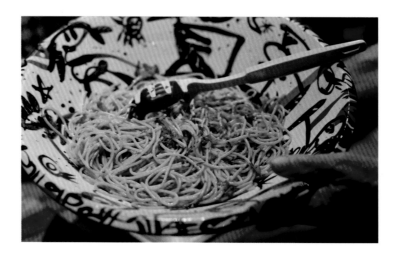

*This pasta with the surprising addition of cinnamon to a savoury sauce appeared in my first cookbook,
Delicious Dishes for Diabetics. I wonder how many were adventurous enough to try it? It does work.
Here it is again in perhaps the more appropriate setting of a vegetarian cookbook. Anna Del Conte says it
comes from Umbria.*

spaghettini with cinnamon and bay leaf tomato sauce

SERVES 4

4 tbsp olive oil

1 large onion, chopped

450g/1lb tomatoes, chopped, with some of their juice

¼ tsp ground cinnamon

10 bay leaves

400g/14oz wholewheat spaghettini

salt and freshly ground black pepper

1 Heat the oil in a large frying pan over a medium to low. Add the onion and sauté for 10 minutes, until softened but not browned.

2 Add the tomatoes, cinnamon and bay. Season well with salt and pepper and cook gently for about 20 minutes, to form a thickish sauce.

3 Cook the pasta in a large saucepan of salted water according to your taste or the packet instructions. Reserve a few large spoonfuls of the pasta cooking water, then drain.

4 Transfer the pasta to the frying pan, adding a couple of tablespoons of the cooking water. Mix well and cook over a gentle heat for 1–2 minutes. This is usually served without cheese – but that's up to you.

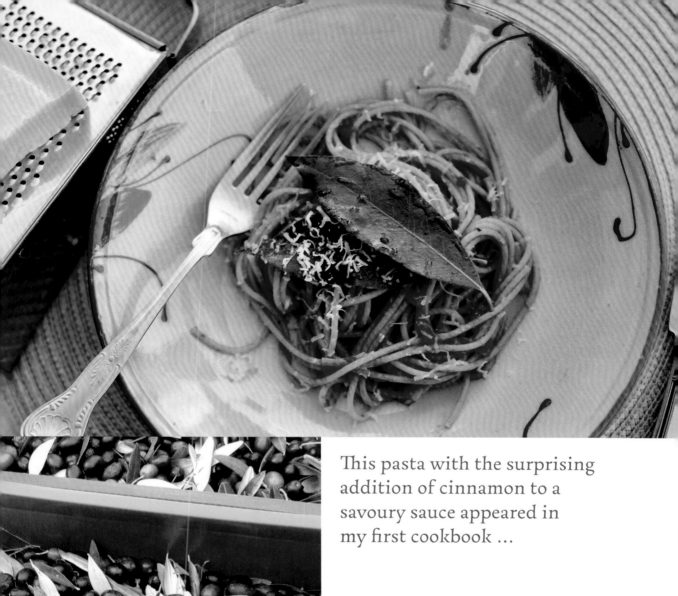

This pasta with the surprising addition of cinnamon to a savoury sauce appeared in my first cookbook …

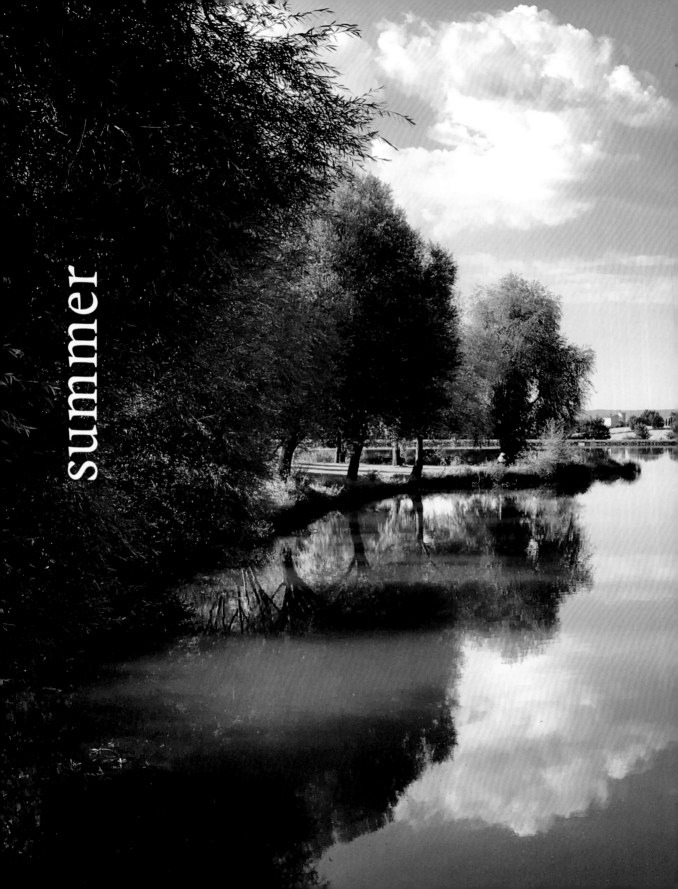

summer

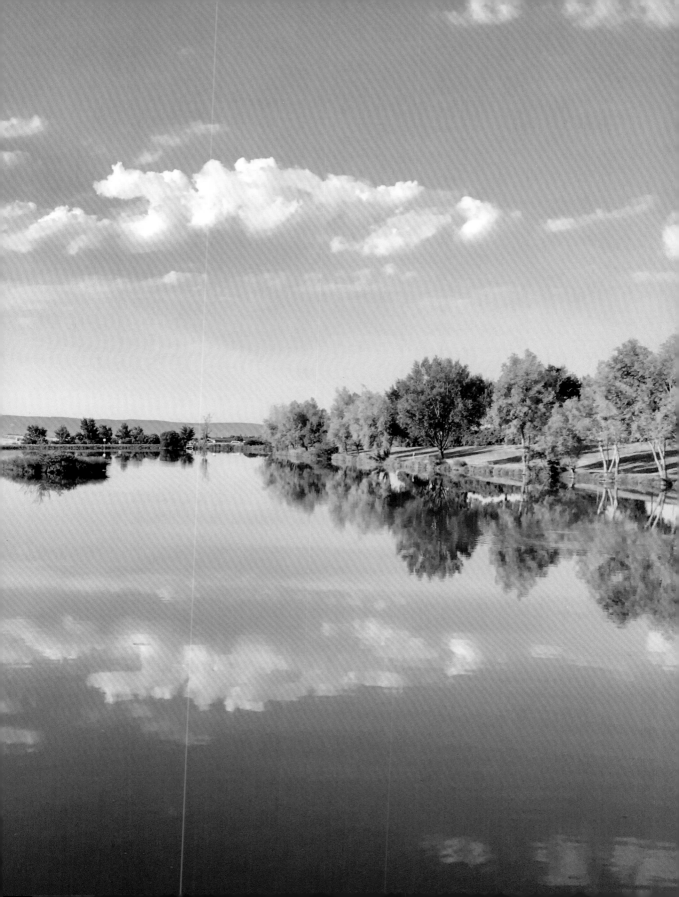

> 'Summer cooking implies a sense of immediacy, a capacity to capture the essence of the fleeting moment.'
>
> Elizabeth David

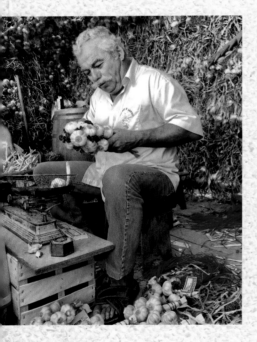

Summer is festival (*fête*) time. Every village has at least one – some in celebration of a particular product associated with that place. In Lautrec it's the garlic festival – La Fête de l'Ail Rose de Lautrec (festival of pink garlic) – on the first Friday and Saturday in August. Ten thousand people squeeze through the narrow streets of this thirteenth-century village, stopping in the main square at noon for a bowl of *soupe à l'ail* – compliments of the mayor.

There's a prize for the best model made with garlic – Loch Ness monsters, Notre Dames, World Cups and Penny Farthings have featured. On the back of a farm truck, laid out like a stable, *paysans* (smallholders) demonstrate the art of trussing garlic and chat amiably with the passing multitude. A parade of Confréries – guilds representing artisan skills practised all over the southwest – snakes languidly round the village led by a traditional jazz band. Men and women dressed in heavy medieval costumes carry banners of the cheese makers, pork butchers, wine makers, bakers – no candlestick makers as yet – and make their way in the midday sun to the open-air theatre on the ramparts, where new members of the Confrérie de l'Ail Rose de Lautrec are solemnly sworn in.

In the evening the boules arena, just outside the village, is the setting for a Grand Repas. Long lines of trestle tables are set up and a simple meal of charcuterie and *confit de canard* is efficiently served to a thousand people – no vegetarian alternative on offer here!

We sit and talk with strangers as the sun slowly relents and slips into the Pyrenees, three hours' drive to the southwest of us.

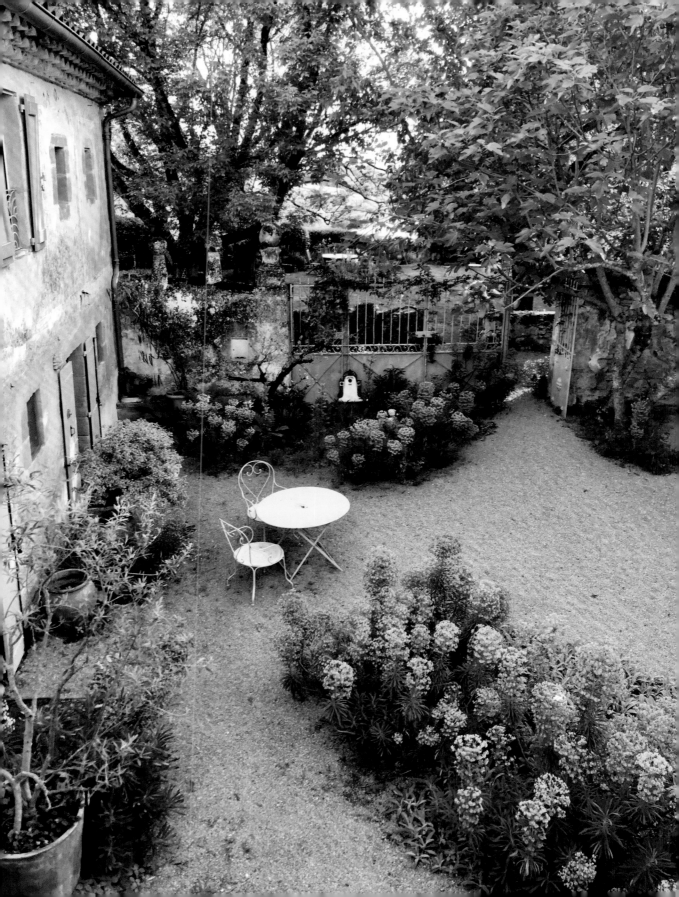

This classic soup first appeared in my second cookbook, Healthy Eating for Life. It is a regular at lunches in the garden in August. Delicious and simple to make, it requires no cooking at all. I include it again in memory of my mother, whose cooking inspired me to get in the kitchen. This is what I wrote then: 'It's a fair bet my mother first tasted this traditional summer soup from Andalusia in 1953, when my parents took my brother and me to the Costa Brava for a fortnight's holiday. Dad worked for British Railways and got a certain amount of concessionary travel in Europe. There were five hotels in Lloret de Mar (500+ now!).

ma's gazpacho

SERVES 8

1kg/2lb 4oz ripe tomatoes, roughly chopped, juice reserved

½ large cucumber, peeled and roughly diced

½ large red pepper, deseeded and roughly diced

2 spring onions, chopped

3 garlic cloves, pulped in a mortar with 1 tsp salt

3 tbsp red wine vinegar

2 tbsp olive oil, plus extra to serve

a few drops of Tabasco (optional)

salt and freshly ground black pepper

a few parsley or basil leaves (optional), chopped, to serve

8 ice cubes (optional), to serve

1 Put the tomatoes, cucumber, red pepper, spring onions and garlic in a food processor. Pulse to combine until you have a not-too-smooth. Tip the purée mixture into a large bowl and season with salt and pepper.

2 Stir in the red wine vinegar and olive oil and add a few drops of Tabasco if you wish – it's a matter of taste. Chill for a couple of hours or overnight.

3 When you're ready to serve, pour a ladleful of the gazpacho into each bowl, add a whirl of olive oil and a pinch of chopped parsley or basil, if you wish. I sometimes add an ice cube to each bowl, too.

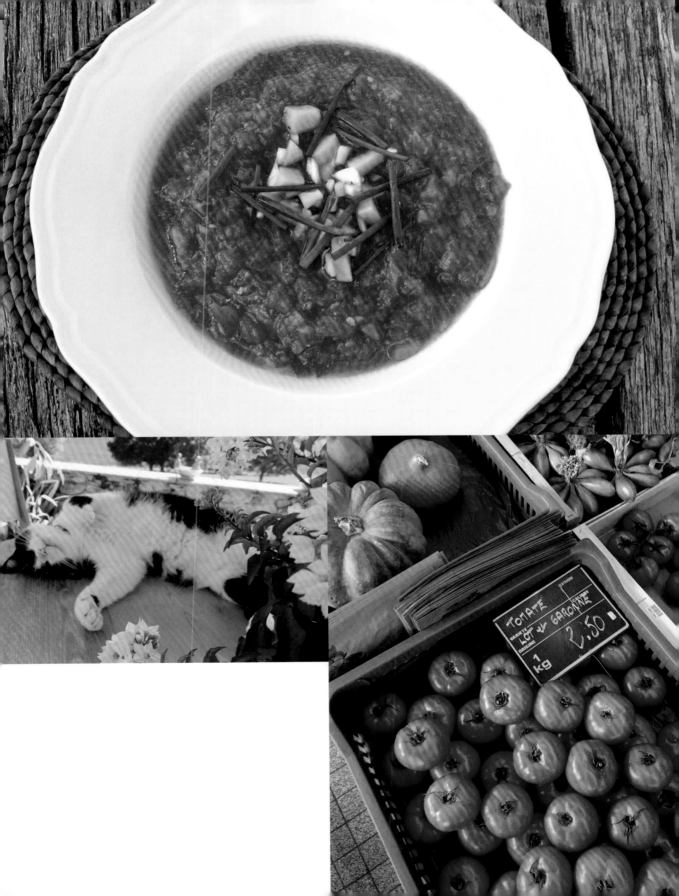

This little dish is a speciality on Milos (one of the Cyclades group of Greek islands and where the Venus de Milo was found). It is very simple and transports you to a table at a quayside restaurant facing the sparkling Aegean Sea. There are two ways to cook it: in a medium-sized shallow terracotta dish or in a foil parcel. I chose the former.

bouyiourdi, baked feta with tomatoes

SERVES 2, AT A STRETCH!

2 ripe tomatoes, sliced

1 red or sweet onion, sliced into half moons

1 chilli, finely chopped, or a couple of pinches of chilli flakes

a couple of pinches of dried oregano

2 tbsp olive oil

100g/3½oz feta cheese

freshly ground black pepper

1 Preheat the oven to 200°C/400°F.

2 Lay half the tomato and onion slices evenly over the base of a small oven dish and sprinkle over half the chilli, a pinch of oregano and half the olive oil. Season with a couple of grindings of pepper.

3 Lay the feta on top and then add a second layer of tomato and onions, sprinkled with chilli and olive oil and seasoned with black pepper.

4 Bake in the top of the oven for about 25 minutes. It should be sizzling but not burnt, so best to check it after 20 minutes.

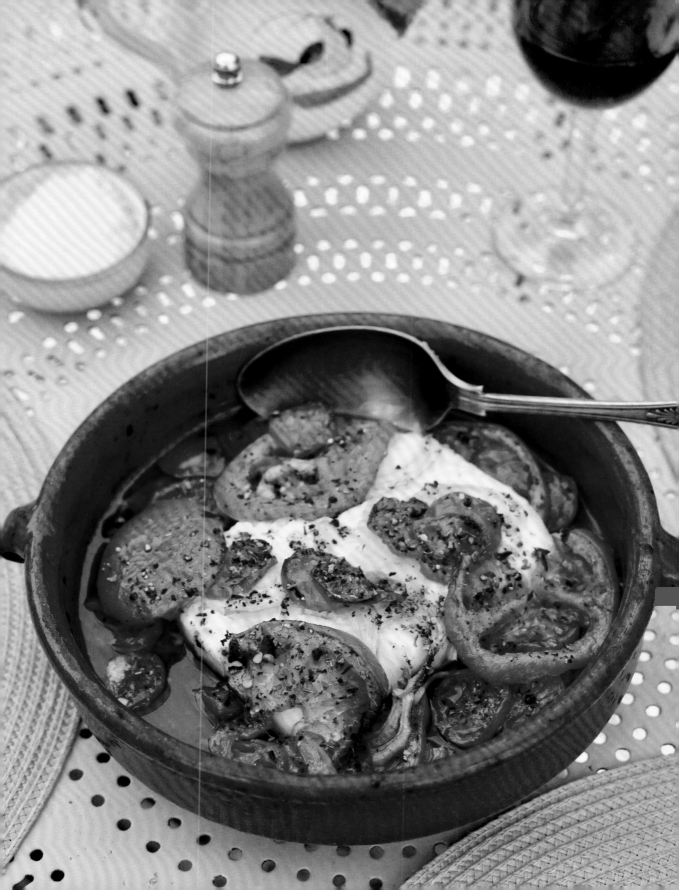

I first encountered this simple, elegant starter at the lunch bar of the veggie section of Eataly – the vast food emporium on 5th and 23rd Street in Manhattan. It looked so cool I had to have it. The beans were stiletto thin and had barely seen boiling water. They were a touch too crunchy. Here less so, but they still retain a bite. I eat them with my fingers, one by one.

crunchy green beans with roasted almonds and lemon zest

SERVES 4

225g/8oz fine green beans

4 tbsp olive oil

100g/⅔ cup almonds, roasted and sliced

zest of 1 or 2 lemons

a bunch of chives, left whole

salt

1 Plunge the beans into salted boiling water for 2–3 minutes, depending on how al dente you like them. Then, quickly run them under cold water to stop them cooking further. Dry them thoroughly in kitchen paper and put them in a bowl.

2 Pour over the olive oil, season with a little salt, and turn the beans to coat.

3 Divide the bean mixture equally between four plates. Sprinkle over the almonds and lemon zest just before serving. Add a few chives to the top, to complement the look.

Glorious new season garlic with glorious new season green beans (they should snap eagerly when you bend them) and the best olive oil you can find!

In Lautrec, the new batch of garlic is celebrated on the first Friday and Saturday of August (see p. 66) – and it's a glorious couple of days!

green beans with garlic

SERVES 4

400g/14oz best-quality green beans

2–3 tbsp olive oil

1 garlic clove, crushed with a
pinch of salt

salt

1 Put a pan of salted water on to boil. Once boiling, add the beans and cook until just tender. Drain them and tip them into a bowl.

2 Pour over the oil, season with a good pinch of salt and add the garlic. Mix thoroughly before serving.

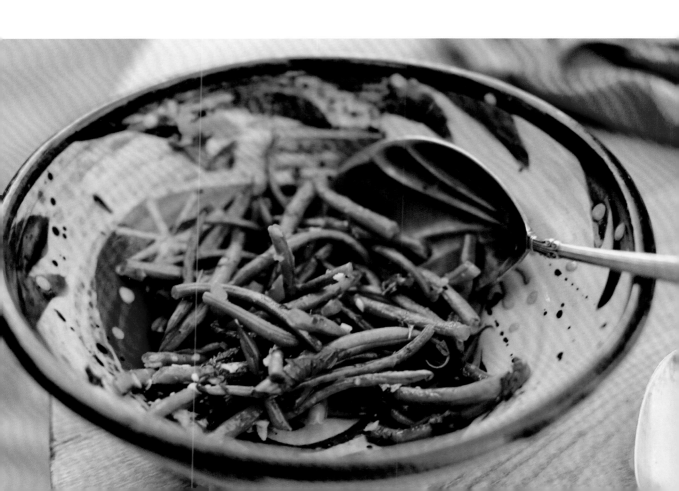

Sweet and savoury. Our friend Helen Richmond tipped us the wink on this unusual combo. The tang of the lime juice offsets the sweetness of the melon. The mild bite of the onion complements the saltiness of the feta. The colours are seductive. I shut my eyes as I take a mouthful and I'm back on holiday in Corfu. Thank you, Helen!

watermelon salad

SERVES 8 AS A STARTER

1.5kg/3½lb watermelon (unpeeled weight)

a good handful of juicy pitted black olives, halved

250g/9oz feta cheese, cut into small dice

1 small red onion, finely sliced

a handful of mint leaves, chopped

2 tbsp lime juice

6 tbsp olive oil

a handful of flat-leaf parsley, leaves picked

freshly ground black pepper

1 Release the flesh of the melon by carefully running a sharp knife round the inside of the crescent of rind – take your time! Lightly steer a teaspoon along the ridge of pips, skilfully dislodging them without mushing up the flesh. Discard the rind and pips and cut the flesh into bite-sized dice.

2 Place the melon and the olives in a bowl and add the feta. Sprinkle over the red onion and the mint.

3 In a separate bowl, mix together the lime juice, olive oil and a couple of grinds of black pepper. (Alternatively, a screw-top jar is good for this: just add your ingredients and shake it all about!) Pour the dressing over the salad, then carefully turn the salad to coat.

4 Top with the parsley leaves and refrigerate until you are ready to serve. This dish is best served thoroughly chilled.

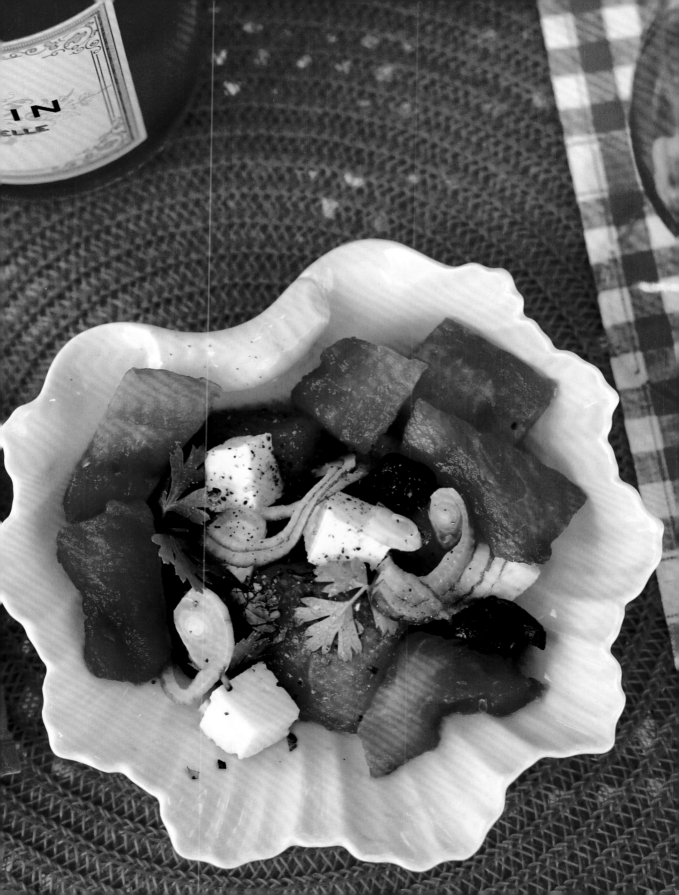

Our friend Theresa, who is a terrific and fearless cook, wrote to say she made this for lunch on a hot day. Served under the willow tree, it delighted her guests.

If you can find the light green variety of courgette, called romanesco, the effect of light green with yellow is pleasing and inviting. Theresa adds grated Parmesan. My version has a Greek slant with strips of black olives – the best you can find – and crumblings of feta. A fine swivel peeler is perfect for slicing the courgettes for this salad.

yellow and green courgette salad

SERVES 4

2 yellow courgettes, sliced into thin ribbons

2 light green courgettes, sliced into thin ribbons

3 tbsp olive oil

1 tbsp lemon juice

a good handful of chives, chopped

a good handful of mint leaves, chopped

6 black olives, sliced into strips

100g/3½oz (approx) feta cheese, crumbled

salt and freshly ground black pepper

1 Place the courgette ribbons in a bowl.

2 In a separate, small bowl, whisk together the oil and lemon juice. Season with salt and pepper and pour the dressing over the courgette ribbons.

3 Add the herbs and the olives to the bowl and crumble over the feta.

4 Park the salad in the fridge until you have laid the table 'under the willow' and are ready to eat lunch.

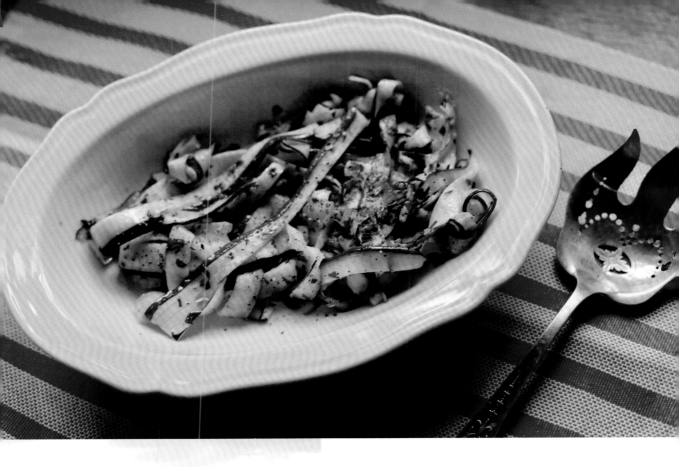

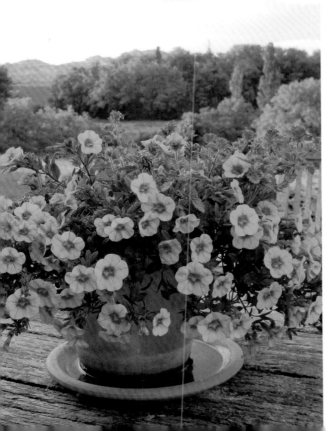

A cool delight on hot days.

Farro is an ancient grain now grown most commonly in the mountainous area of northeast Tuscany. It has a pleasant chewiness and lends itself well to additions of glorious summer stuff. This makes a nice alternative to Salade Niçoise, for example, on a lovely summer's day.

farro summer salad

SERVES 4

For the farro

1 tbsp olive oil

1 small red or sweet onion, finely chopped

450g/1lb farro

1 litre/4 cups vegetable stock

For the summer stuff

3 tbsp olive oil

a good handful of cherry tomatoes, quartered

½ cucumber, peeled, deseeded and diced

1 sweet onion, thinly sliced

1 avocado, finely diced

a good handful of mint leaves and flat-leaf parsley, finely chopped

1 tbsp roasted walnuts, hazelnuts or pistachios, roughly chopped

1 tbsp lemon juice

100g/3½oz feta cheese, crumbled (optional)

salt and freshly ground black pepper

1 Start with the farro. Heat the oil in a pan and gently sauté the onion for 5 minutes to soften but not brown it.

2 Add the farro and turn regularly for 2–3 minutes, to toast it. Add the stock and bring to the boil. Reduce the heat to low, cover the pan and simmer for 15 minutes, until softened but retaining a bit of bite and pleasing crunchiness. Drain and set aside to cool.

3 When you are ready to make the salad, transfer the cooled farro to a serving bowl and add all the summer stuff ingredients, seasoning well with salt and pepper. Carefully fold everything together.

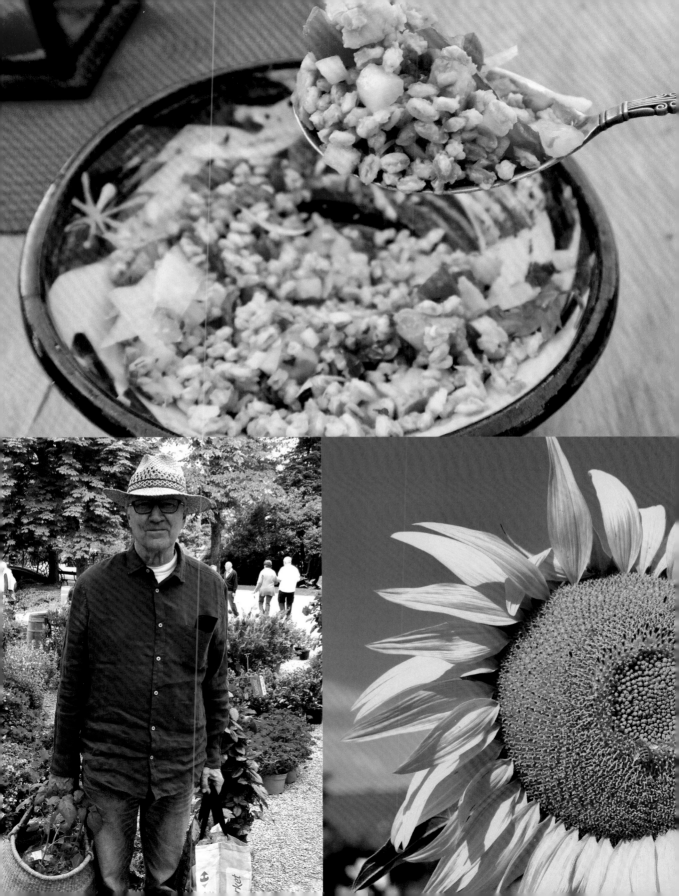

Escalivada is a Catalan salad of roasted vegetables. The name comes from the verb escalivar, *meaning 'to roast in the embers'. I've made this version in the oven, but it's good nonetheless.*

catalan roasted vegetables

SERVES 3 OR 4

1 large sweet onion, unpeeled

2 red peppers

1 yellow pepper

1 aubergine

5 tbsp olive oil

1 tbsp balsamic vinegar

1 garlic clove, chopped

1 tbsp chopped flat-leaf parsley

salt and freshly ground black pepper

1 Preheat the oven to 220°C/425°F.

2 Wrap the onion in foil and put it in a medium baking tray surrounded by the other whole vegetables. Sprinkle the vegetables with 2 tablespoons of the olive oil and season generously with salt, then roast in the upper part of the oven for 1 hour or until the pepper and aubergine skins are charred and loosened.

3 Using kitchen tongs transfer the peppers and aubergine to a plastic bag to sweat and cool – taking care not to lose the cooking juices, as these will form part of the dressing later.

4 When they are cool enough to handle, take the vegetables out of the bag. Remove the loosened skins and seeds from the peppers and the skin of the aubergine – again taking care to keep the juices.

5 Slice the skinned peppers and aubergine lengthways and place side by side on a serving dish.

6 Unwrap the onion from the foil and cut it in half. Slice each half and lay them next to the peppers and aubergine.

7 Pour the juices from the bag into a mixing bowl and add the balsamic vinegar and the remaining olive oil. Whisk together to make a dressing and pour it over the vegetables. Stir in the garlic and parsley and… *Gaudeix* (Catalan for enjoy)!

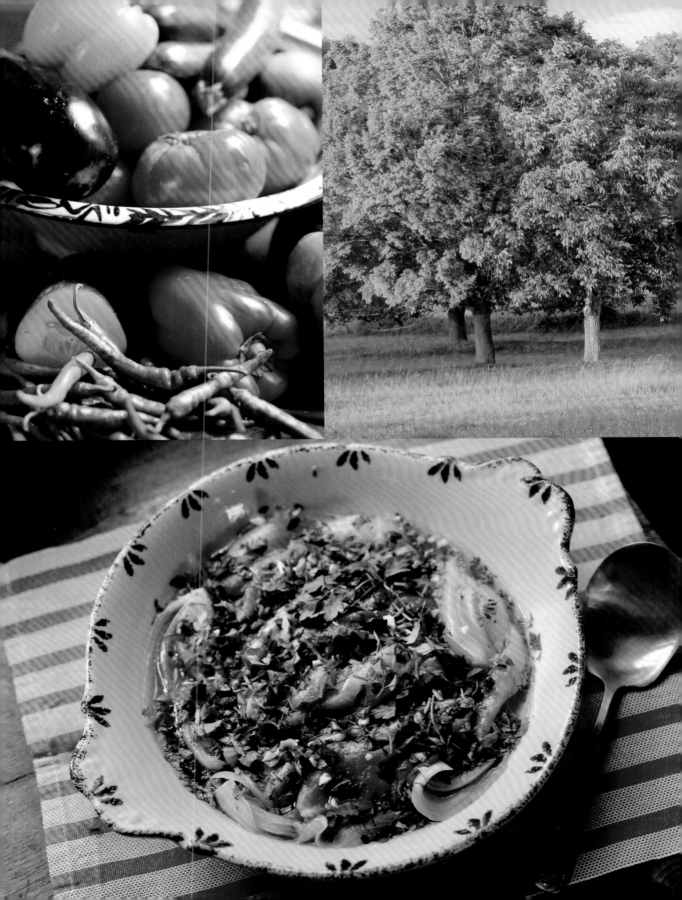

Messy but marvellous, this simple summer salad displays the colours of Catalonia, the historic region just to the southeast of us that, like the Basque Country in the west, pays no heed to the national borders of France and Spain.

red and yellow pepper salad

SERVES 4

3 large red peppers

1 yellow pepper

olive oil

salt and freshly ground black pepper

1 Preheat the oven to 240°C/465°F.

2 Place all the peppers in a baking tray and roast for 20 minutes, turning halfway through cooking – this will result in the skins being nicely charred.

3 Set the peppers aside to cool down. This is the messy bit. When they have cooled, carefully peel off the skins, slit them open and remove the seeds and pith. (It's so satisfying when you manage to lift a large piece of skin in one piece. Take your time and enjoy the messiness!)

4 The peppers will break down into pieces as you peel. Lay the pieces on a pretty plate, season with salt and pepper and dress with a sprinkling of olive oil.

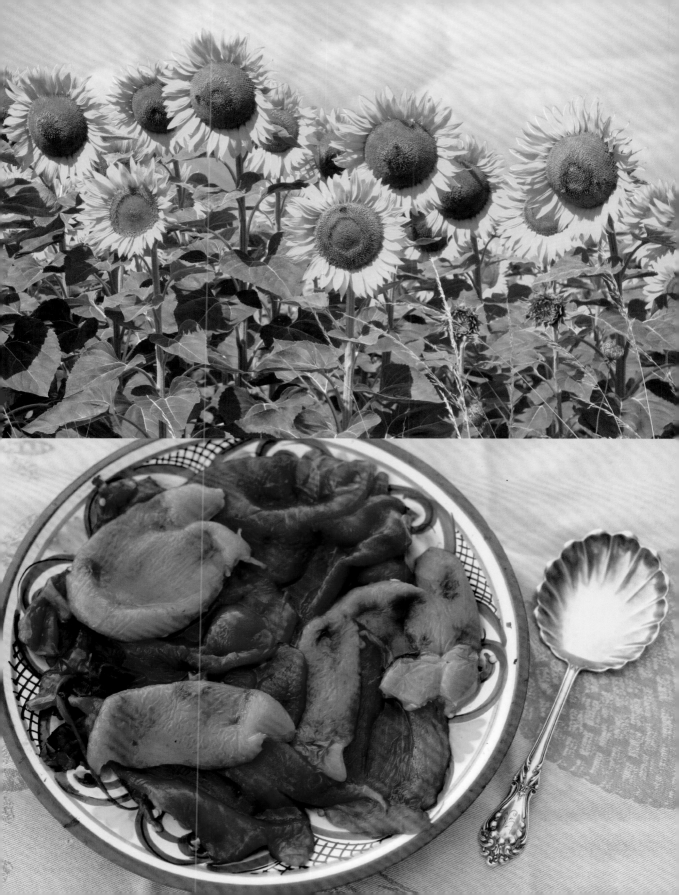

A light lunch and a cousin of my Leftover Pasta with Eggs (see p.92)

eggs with ripe tomatoes

SERVES 1

1 tbsp olive oil

1 onion, roughly chopped

2 tomatoes, sliced thick

1 garlic clove, chopped

2 eggs

salt and freshly ground black pepper

rye bread, toasted (optional), to serve

1 Heat the olive oil in a medium saucepan and soften the onion over a medium–low heat for 5 minutes.

2 Add the tomatoes, then season with salt and pepper and add the garlic. Cook for a further 5 minutes, until the garlic has softened, then carefully turn the mixture over and break two eggs into the pan.

3 Cover the pan and allow the eggs to set before seasoning to taste and sliding onto a plate to serve. I allow myself a slice of rye toast to soak up the sauce.

This is high summer fare. Large variety tomatoes sliced satisfyingly into thick rounds make a simple and easy-to-do lunch on a hot day and can be served with a simple green salad.

large tomato steaks topped with pecorino and feta

SERVES 2

olive oil

2 large tomatoes, cut into 1cm/½in-thick rounds

½ tbsp grated pecorino or Parmesan per tomato

½ tbsp crumbled feta cheese per tomato

salt (remembering that feta is salty) and freshly ground black pepper

2 thin slices of wholemeal or rye bread toast, to serve

1 Preheat the oven to 180°C/350°F.

2 Lay a sheet of foil on a baking tray and brush with olive oil. Lay the tomato slices on the foil, drizzle with olive oil and lightly season with salt and pepper.

3 Sprinkle over the grated pecorino or Parmesan and the feta. Drizzle again with a little olive oil, then bake in the top of the oven for about 20 minutes, until the tomatoes are completely tender, with the cheese pleasingly browned on top.

4 Toast the bread, drizzle with olive oil and serve.

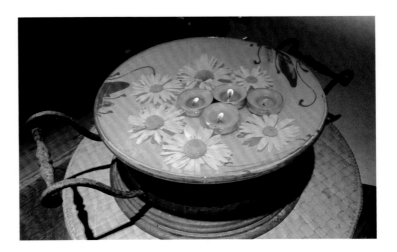

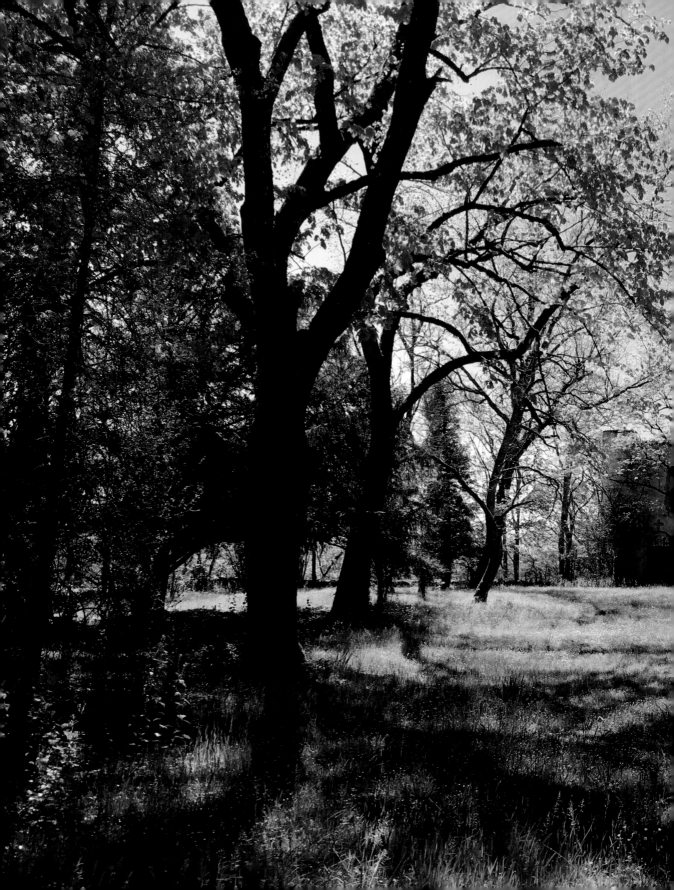

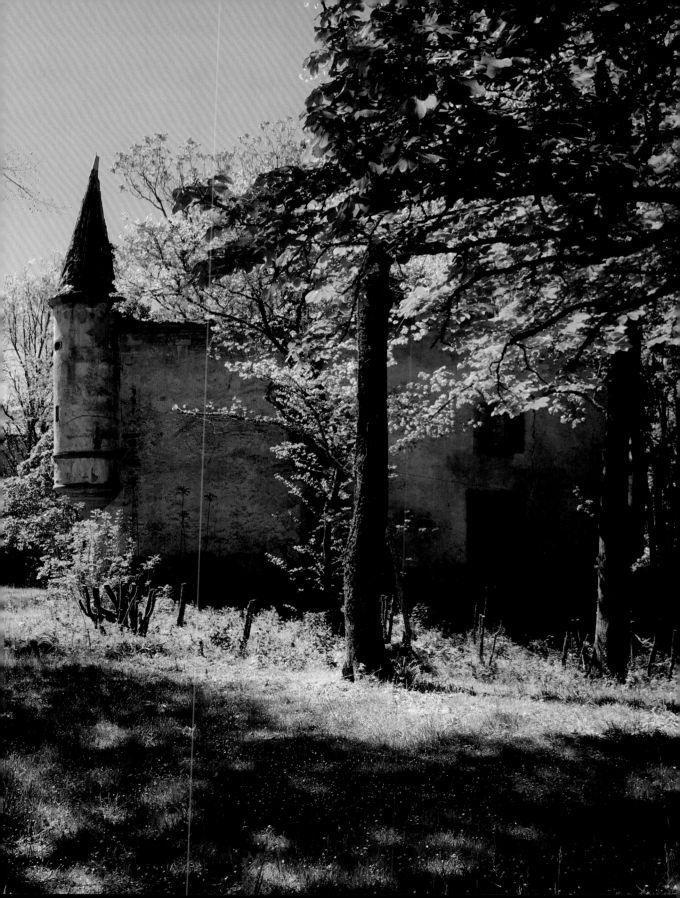

This enigmatic, gentle giant of a vegetable goes by many names, depending on where you're from – aubergine, eggplant, melanzane. A tortino is a sort of soufflé crossed with a no-pastry pie – handy for those who need to watch their intake of refined carbohydrates. It's a little labour intensive but pays off. This tortino recipe is adapted from one in Paola Gavin's Italian Vegetarian Cooking. You'll need to begin by draining the aubergine for at least 1 hour before you intend to cook.

aubergine tortino

SERVES 4

700g/1½lb aubergine, peeled and
thinly sliced

olive oil

50g/2oz Parmesan, grated

70g/12½oz tomato sauce (see p.211)

5 eggs

salt and freshly ground black pepper

1 Lightly salt the aubergine slices and leave them to drain in a colander for at least 1 hour.

2 Once drained, dry the slices in between sheets of kitchen paper.

3 Preheat the oven to 190°C/375°F.

4 Oil a couple of shallow oven trays. Lightly brush the aubergine slices with olive oil and lay them out in a single layer on the trays. Bake for 5 minutes on each side on the top shelf of the oven, one tray at a time.

5 Heat a cast-iron griddle pan to hot. Transfer the slices onto the griddle pan and char them for 2–3 minutes on each side. The grilling adds a smoky flavour; you could fry the slices or just leave them in the oven longer, but they must cook until they are tender.

6 Oil a shallow oven dish and layer the aubergine slices in the bottom.

7 In a bowl, mix together the cheese and the tomato sauce and season with salt and pepper.

8 In a separate bowl, whisk the eggs and stir them into the cheese and tomato mixture. Pour this over the aubergine slices, to cover. Bake in the middle of the oven for 20–25 minutes until the dish is lightly browned on top.

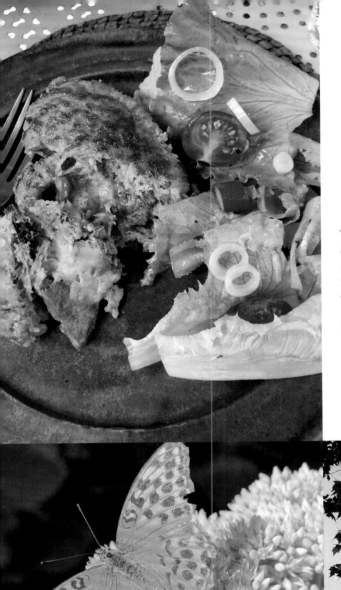

A tortino is a sort of soufflé crossed with a no-pastry pie – handy for those who need to watch their intake of refined carbohydrates.

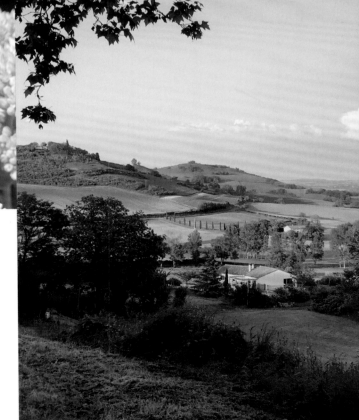

According to Alan Davidson's wonderful Oxford Companion to Food, ratatouille is a relatively recent creation. The word, which comes from the French touiller, to stir, first pops up in 1877, misspelled, in reference to a meat stew. It is not until the 1930s that it becomes associated with a 'ragout of aubergine with tomatoes, courgettes and sweet pepper'.

The defining quality of summer food is colour. The stands at markets are bursting with it, blindingly so. Here is colour in abundance and it makes my heart sing.

my ratatouille for two

SERVES 2

2 tbsp olive oil

2 onions, halved and halved again and sliced

2 garlic cloves, roughly chopped

2 red peppers, deseeded and cut into rough squares

1 yellow pepper, deseeded and cut into rough squares

a handful of small green peppers, if you can find them, deseeded and cut into rough squares

1 small fresh or dried red chilli, finely chopped

1 tsp coriander seeds, crushed

400g ripe tomatoes, roughly chopped, juice reserved

salt and freshly ground black pepper

1 Heat half the oil in a shallow pan on a gentle heat, add the onions and sweat for 10 minutes until softened. Add the garlic and cook for a further 2 minutes, then add the remaining oil, along with the peppers, chilli and coriander seeds. Stir well.

2 Cover the pan and cook over a low heat for 10 minutes, until the peppers have softened and lost their hard bite. Add the chopped tomatoes (reserving the juice) to the pan, season well with salt and pepper and stir everything together.

3 Cook until the tomatoes have integrated with the peppers to make a delicious summer sauce. Add a little of the reserved tomato juice as the tomatoes cook, if necessary, but this version should not be too mushy.

4 Serve with a dollop of tapenade (see p.212) or pesto (see p.207) and some green beans with garlic (see p.73).

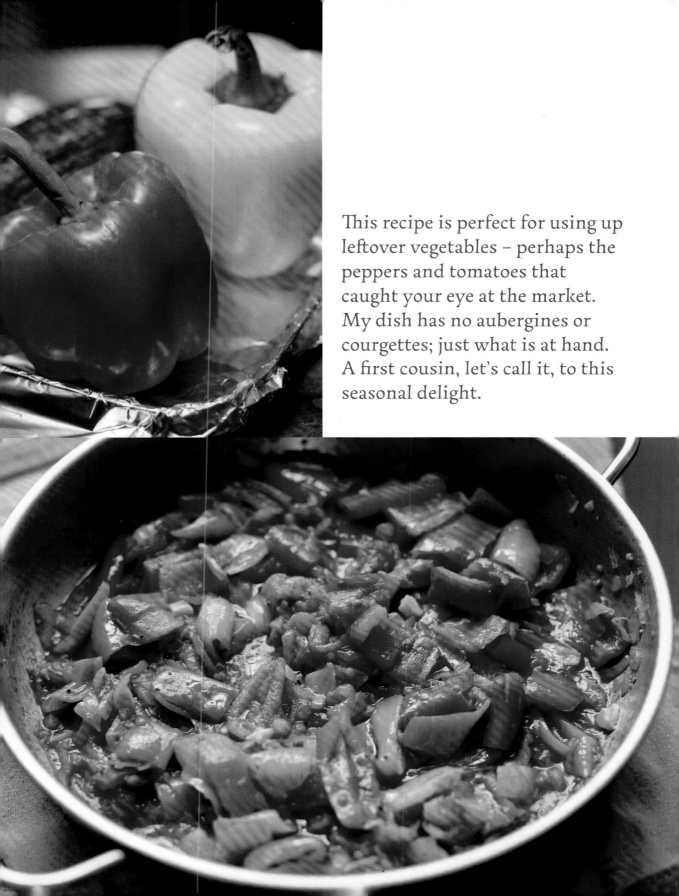

This recipe is perfect for using up leftover vegetables – perhaps the peppers and tomatoes that caught your eye at the market. My dish has no aubergines or courgettes; just what is at hand. A first cousin, let's call it, to this seasonal delight.

Sunday night is pasta night here – a once-a-week treat and, to be honest, a night off from thinking about what to cook. I allow 225g/8oz of pasta between the two of us, so there is usually some left over to reheat for this tasty lunch. This is nice, oily stuff, made with spaghettini or penne as a rule. It stays in the fridge until I notice it on Tuesday and rejoice!

leftover pasta with eggs

SERVES 2

leftover cooked pasta
(from the fridge)

4 eggs

salt and freshly ground black pepper

1 Empty the leftover pasta into a frying pan and reheat it over a low heat, turning occasionally as it begins to brown and caramelise a little – about 20 minutes.

2 Crack 4 eggs into a bowl and spread them carefully on top of the pasta.

3 Cover the pan and cook for about 5 minutes, then check to see if the eggs are done to your liking. Separate the mix in two and, using a fish slice, lift onto separate plates. Season to taste and there you have a lazy Tuesday lunch – served with a green salad, perhaps.

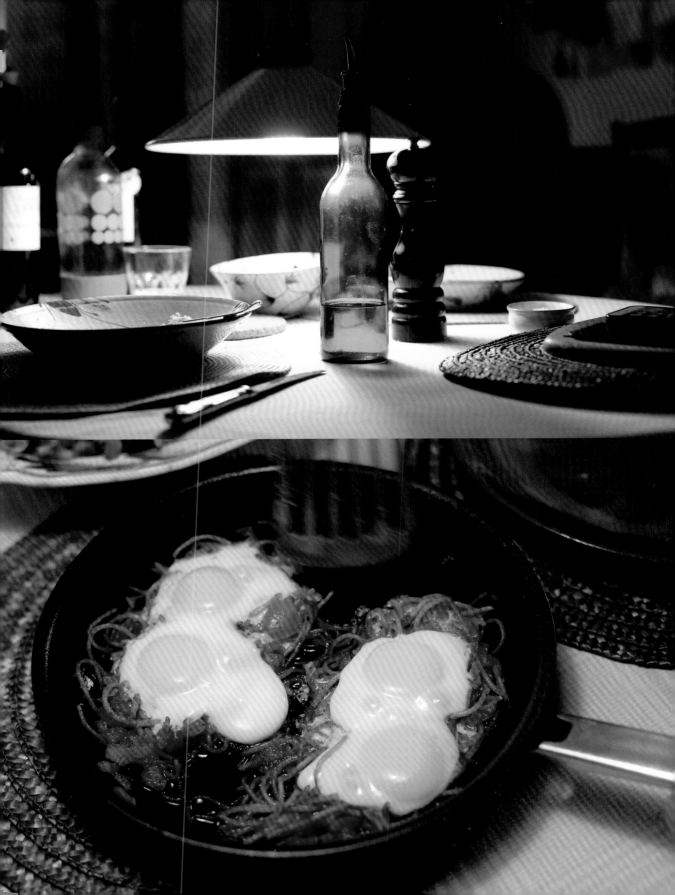

This is a stew with summer in its DNA. It has enough comfort factor to lift the spirits, even if you eat it at a point in the summer when the seasonal sweetness of fresh tomatoes is not yet fully expressed.

It's inspired by a Martha Rose Shulman recipe in the New York Times. Few ingredients, simple to make and a pleasing look – just the ticket!

courgette and bean stew

SERVES 3 OR 4

2 tbsp olive oil

1 onion, chopped

3 garlic cloves, pulped with ½ tsp of salt

3 medium courgettes, sliced into 1cm/½in rounds

250g/9oz chopped tomatoes (fresh or tinned)

250g/9oz cherry tomatoes, halved

3 thyme sprigs

250g/9oz good-quality cooked white beans (tinned or from a jar)

salt and freshly ground black pepper

1 Heat the oil in a medium saucepan over a medium–low heat and add the onion. Sweat for 5–7 minutes until softened, then add the garlic and sauté for a few seconds, taking care not to let it burn.

2 Add the courgettes and turn them over in the mixture. Cook for about 5 minutes, until they start to soften, then add all the tomatoes, the thyme sprigs and a seasoning of salt and pepper. Cook for 10 minutes, until the cherry tomatoes start to soften.

3 Add the beans and their liquid or a couple of tablespoons of water. Cook for a further 15 minutes, until it has settled into an inviting sauce. Season with salt and pepper to taste.

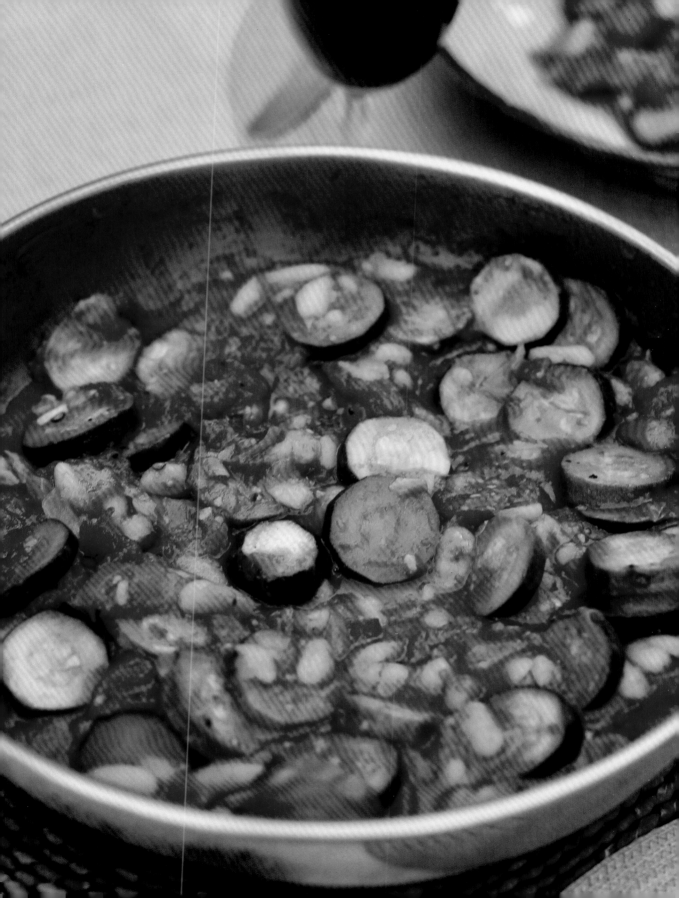

This has been on our menu for years. The combinations in this classic Italian frittata depend on slow cooking the onions in the first stage and the frittata itself later on – the point of a frittata (and what sets it apart from a French omelette) is that it takes time – if you cook it too fast it will dry out.

It's a good dish for when you have company – you can cook it beforehand and serve it at room temperature. It tastes even better the next day.

courgette and onion frittata

SERVES 4

4 tbsp olive oil

3 onions, thinly sliced in a food processor

3 courgettes, thinly sliced in a food processor

5 large eggs, beaten

50g/2oz Parmesan, grated

salt and freshly ground black pepper

1 Heat the oil in a large frying pan over a low heat and add the onions. Cook, turning occasionally, for 35–40 minutes, until nicely coloured, soft and caramelised. This step will take the longest. The longer you cook the onions, the sweeter they will taste and the less likely the frittata will dry out. (You can cook on medium heat, turning more often, and half the cooking time, if you prefer, but I think the best results come from taking things slowly.)

2 Add the sliced courgettes and a pinch of salt. Turn the mixture over thoroughly and cook over a medium heat for about 7 minutes, until the courgettes are soft.

3 Remove the pan from the heat and push the mixture to one side of the pan. Slip something under that side of the pan to prop it up at a slight angle so that the oily cooking liquid drains away from the mixture to the empty side of the pan. Leave to cool in this way for 10 minutes or so, then scoop out the drained oil and put it in a small bowl.

4 Place the beaten eggs into a large bowl. Add the cooled courgette and onion mixture, then stir to combine and season to taste. Fold in the Parmesan.

5 Heat a tablespoon of the oil you set aside in a frying pan (about 26cm/10½in diameter) with an ovenproof handle. Pour in the eggy mixture and cook over the lowest possible heat for about 30 minutes – until there is only a small puddle of the mixture left on top. Meanwhile, heat the grill to hot.

6 Slip the pan under the grill for 1–2 minutes, lightly browning the top of the frittata. Remove from the grill. Ease a spatula round the circumference of the pan and gingerly under the frittata. When you sense the frittata is free from the pan base, ease it out of the pan and on to a serving plate.

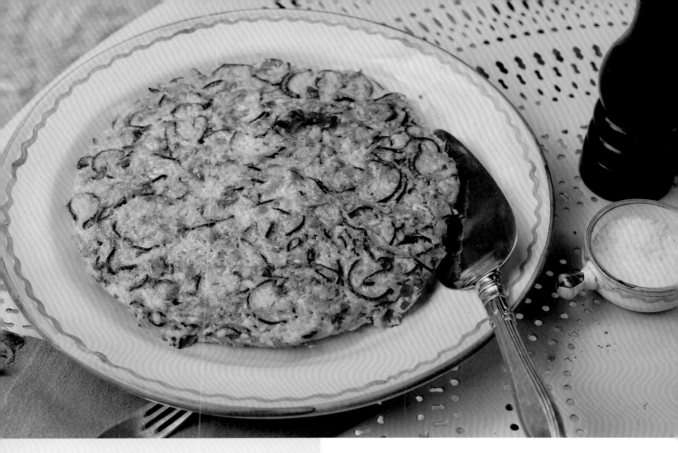

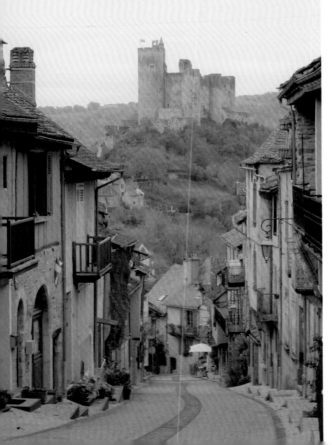

It's a good dish for when you have company – you can cook it beforehand and serve it at room temperature. It tastes even better the next day.

I was scrabbling around for a starter to serve at the Garlic Festival lunch when I noticed three aubergines sitting looking at me expectantly. The idea for rounds came from Antonio Carluccio's Vegetables cookbook. You'll need to salt them for at least 1 hour before you intend to cook.

aubergine rounds with tomato slices and feta

SERVES 2

1 largish aubergine, sliced into
1cm/½in rounds

olive oil

a large handful of fresh basil, parsley
and mint, chopped together

150g/5oz feta cheese, crumbled

2 ripe tomatoes, sliced into rounds

1 tbsp grated Parmesan per slice

salt and freshly ground black pepper

1 Salt the aubergine slices and leave them to drain in a colander for at least 1 hour.

2 Preheat the oven to 220°C/425°F. Line a baking tray with foil and brush it with a little olive oil.

3 Dry the aubergine rounds with kitchen paper. Brush both sides with olive oil and lay them out evenly on the baking tray. Bake in the top of the oven for 20–25 minutes, until thoroughly cooked and soft.

4 Stir together the chopped herbs and the feta in a bowl and, using a teaspoon, spread a little on each cooked aubergine round.

5 Lay a tomato slice on each aubergine round and sprinkle with a pinch of salt and a little olive oil. Top them off with a tablespoon of grated Parmesan.

6 Return the tray to the top of the oven and cook the stacked aubergine slices for a further 15–20 minutes, until the tomato has a melted look and the Parmesan has browned a little.

7 Serve them straightaway or at room temperature.

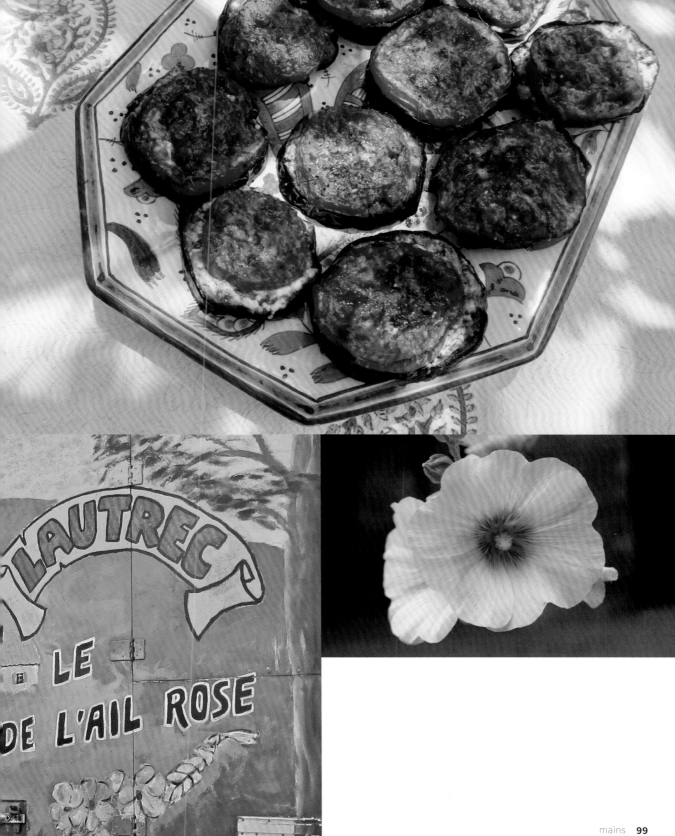

The clue is in the name. There's a trend to ape steaks with juicy slices of vegetables. Here, thick slices of ripe tomato are topped with a mini Greek salad – a few black olives, a little chopped cucumber, red onion and some crumbled feta – to make a starter or light lunch. You'll need a sharp knife and keen eye.

raw beefsteak tomato steaks

SERVES 4

1 or 2 large ripe tomatoes, sliced into 2cm/¾in-thick slices

½ cucumber, deseeded and diced

½ small red onion, diced

12 juicy pitted black olives, roughly chopped

150g/5oz feta cheese, crumbled

4 tbsp olive oil

salt and freshly ground black pepper

4 basil leaves, to serve

1 Choose the four best slices of tomato (dice the rest and set aside to add to the mini salad). Place a slice of tomato on each of four plates (choose plates to offset the colour, if you can). Season with a little salt and a turn of the pepper mill.

2 Add equal amounts of cucumber, red onion, olives, feta and diced tomato on top of the tomato slices. Finish with a drizzle of olive oil and serve topped with a basil leaf.

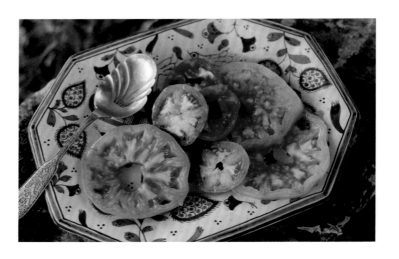

The brightest colours are not showing yet – tomatoes, red peppers – but include a yellow courgette in the mix and the hint is there.

You'll need to begin salting the vegetables a couple of hours or the night before you intend to cook.

aubergine, courgette and green pepper sauté

SERVES 4 AS A SIDE

1 large aubergine, peeled and chopped into 2cm/¾in pieces

1 yellow courgette, chopped into 2cm/¾in pieces

1 green courgette, chopped into 2cm/¾in pieces

3 tbsp olive oil, plus extra for drizzlin

1 green pepper, deseeded and chopped into 4cm/1½in squares

1 tbsp rosemary needles, chopped very fine

1 tsp fennel seeds, finely chopped

1 garlic clove, finely chopped

½ tsp chilli flakes

1 lemon, halved, for squeezing

salt and freshly ground black pepper

1   Salt the chopped aubergine and courgettes separately and leave them to drain through a sieve for a couple of hours or overnight. I was amazed this morning how much liquid had drained off. Give them a squeeze and dry them thoroughly.

2   Heat 2 tablespoons of the oil in a saucepan over a medium–high heat and add the drained aubergine and the green pepper. Sauté for about 7–8 minutes until tender and lightly browned. Add the courgettes and sauté until the courgettes are tender.

3   Mix the rosemary, fennel, garlic and chilli with the remaining olive oil in a small bowl. Stir the mixture into the pan with the vegetables, turning everything to coat thoroughly. Cook for 5 minutes or more to let the flavours develop and the vegetables soften thoroughly. Check the seasoning, squeeze the lemon over and drizzle with a little more olive oil before serving.

An early summer treat.

For a wintry alternative, check out the Simple Spicy Winter Vegetable Stew on p.189. The two stews illustrate how effortlessly fresh vegetables can work together to produce tasty results. Put together the right cast and a well-written play barely needs a director. This is straightforward, but has lovely subtle aromas. As it cooks, they beckon.

simple summer stew

SERVES 3 OR 4

1 aubergine, peeled and diced

1 courgette, diced

3 tbsp olive oil, plus extra to serve

1 onion, chopped

1 garlic clove, pulped in a mortar

1 tsp fennel seeds, roughly mashed

4 tomatoes, peeled, deseeded and chopped

1 fennel bulb, outer layers removed, halved and diced

½ sweet potato, peeled and diced

200g/7oz tinned chickpeas, drained

250ml/1 cup vegetable stock

salt and freshly ground black pepper

a handful of flat-leaf parsley, chopped, to serve

1 Sprinkle the diced aubergine and courgette with salt and leave them to drain in a sieve for an hour or more. Once drained, squeeze them and dry them with kitchen paper.

2 Heat 2 tablespoons of the olive oil in a large, shallow pan (it needs to be big enough to hold all the ingredients) over a medium heat. Add the diced aubergine and courgette and cook for at least 10 minutes, or until browned and softened (the aubergine must be tender – undercooked aubergine is inedible).

3 Add the onion and the remaining olive oil to the pan. Allow the onion to cook for 5 minutes, before adding the garlic and fennel seeds (the garlic needs to soften but be careful not to let it burn). Then add the rest of the vegetables, the chickpeas and the stock. Season with salt and pepper and bring the stock to the boil. Once it's boiling turn the heat down, cover the pan and simmer for about 30 minutes, or until all the vegetables are tender.

4 Serve hot in bowls with a pinch of chopped parsley and a swirl of olive oil.

If you are looking for an alternative to pasta or rice, bulgur wheat is a great option, as it too can be an empty canvas on which to paint your meals.

cooked summer bulgur

SERVES 4

450g/1lb ripe tomatoes, peeled and deseeded

2 tbsp olive oil, plus extra to swirl

½ tsp cayenne pepper

200g/7oz bulgur wheat

salt and freshly ground black pepper

1 Blast the tomatoes to a pulp in a food processor.

2 Heat the oil in a saucepan over a medium heat and add the blitzed tomatoes and the cayenne. Bring up to the boil, turn the heat to low and cook for 10 minutes.

3 Add the bulgur, turn off the heat and let the bulgur absorb the liquid – it will take about 15 minutes.

4 Season with salt and pepper, then stir in a swirl of olive oil before serving.

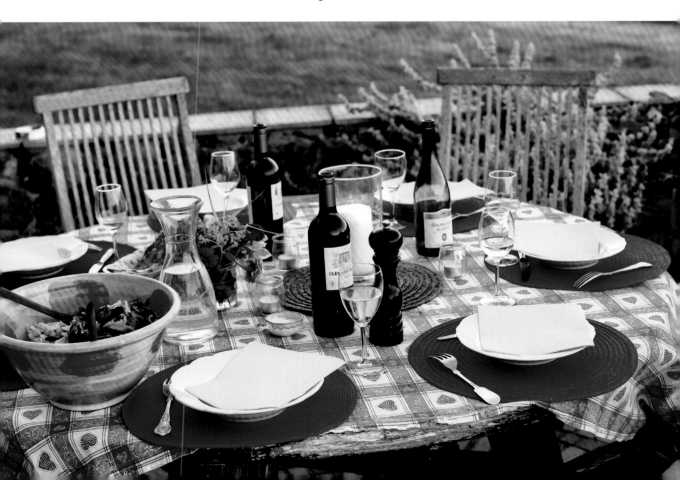

Adapted from Skye Gyngell's version in her book, How I Cook. Featuring new season courgettes, cooked slow with new season garlic and mint, it's a mushily delicious dish with a little kick from the chilli.

slow-cooked courgettes

SERVES 4

1 tbsp olive oil

2 garlic cloves, thinly sliced

1 small dried red chilli, chopped

400g/14oz courgettes, thinly sliced

a handful of mint leaves, chopped

salt and freshly ground black pepper

1 Heat the oil in a medium pan over a low heat. Add the garlic and chilli and cook for 2–3 minutes, until the garlic has softened.

2 Add the sliced courgettes and turn them over in the oil to coat them thoroughly. Season generously with salt and pepper and turn again. Cover the pan and cook for 40 minutes on a very low heat, until the courgettes fall apart. Fold in the mint and serve.

Gorgeously garlicky is all I can say...

quick fried tomato slices with garlic, chilli and parsley

SERVES 4

3 garlic cloves, pulped in a mortar

2 tbsp chopped flat-leaf parsley

1 red chilli, finely chopped

2 tbsp olive oil

450g/1lb ripe tomatoes, thickly sliced

salt and freshly ground black pepper

1 Mix the garlic, parsley and chilli and set aside.

2 Heat the olive oil in a large frying pan over a high heat. Add the tomato slices and fry for 1 minute, seasoning with salt and pepper.

3 Scatter the parsley, garlic and chilli mixture over the slices before turning them over. Season and fry for a further minute. The juices will be running freely and will meld deliciously with whatever else you are serving.

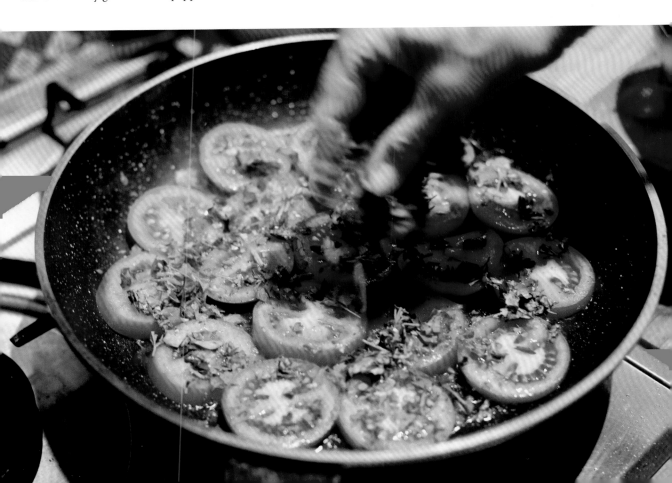

'Cartdriver's spaghettini', this Sicilian pasta dish certainly brightens up a person's day after a long hot haul. It is simple and quick, and often made with uncooked seasonal ingredients, such as garlic, basil and tomatoes. Presumably there were as many versions as there were carts and horses. Here, the sauce is cooked for a short time to allow the hint of chilli heat to kick in and the garlic to meld while retaining the freshness of the ripe tomatoes.

spaghettini carrettiera

SERVES 4

6 tbsp olive oil

6 garlic cloves, finely chopped

a good handful of basil leaves, chopped

1 small red chilli, chopped (with the seeds if you like a hotter version)

700g/1½lb ripe tomatoes, skinned, deseeded and chopped

400g/14oz spaghettini

grated Parmesan, to serve (optional)

olive oil, to serve (optional)

salt and freshly ground black pepper

1 Heat the oil in a medium saucepan. Add all the ingredients except the spaghettini, season to taste, bring to a simmer and cook for 15 minutes. Turn off the heat.

2 Bring a large pan of salted water to the boil and add the pasta. Cook according to the packet instructions or to your taste, then drain and add the sauce, stirring to combine thoroughly.

3 Serve with grated Parmesan if you wish (Meredith did); I was happy with the kick of the garlic and chilli and a swirl of my best olive oil. My word that was tasty!

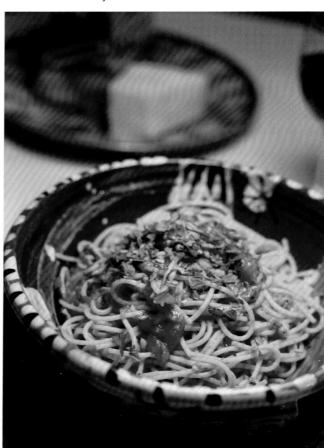

This is something I look forward to every year, not least because it is so quick to make. Our friend Joan sent over parsley and basil from her garden this morning. Both were perfectly fresh, but the parsley was like none I'd ever seen. It shimmered with freshness. This was the only choice for Sunday's regular pasta, even though the tomatoes are not August-ripe yet.

herb-happy spaghettini with raw tomatoes

SERVES 4

1 tbsp mint, chopped

1 tbsp sage, chopped

3 tbsp flat-leaf parsley, chopped

3 tbsp basil, chopped

3 tsp rosemary needles, finely chopped

400g/14oz ripe tomatoes, skinned and roughly chopped

400g/14oz spaghettini

6 tbsp good-quality olive oil

salt and freshly ground black pepper

grated Parmesan, to serve

1 Bring a saucepan of water to the boil and add a teaspoon of salt.

2 Place the chopped herbs in a bowl. Add the chopped tomatoes and season with salt and pepper. Stir carefully to combine.

3 Cook the pasta in the boiling water, according to the packet instructions or to taste. A minute or two before the pasta is ready, heat the olive oil in a small frying pan until it is very hot and pour it over the tomatoes and herbs – the mixture will object with a loud sizzling.

4 Drain the pasta and add it to the bowl. Turn everything over and serve with grated Parmesan.

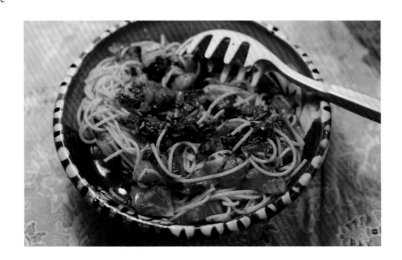

olive oil

When it comes to fat, Mediterranean cooking primarily uses olive oil – the life-blood of this way of eating. To steal an advertising slogan from the sixties for Mackeson, a stout beer: 'It looks good, tastes good and, by golly, it does you good.'

I cook almost exclusively with workaday extra virgin olive oil, i.e. the less expensive, blended types which are now widely available in supermarkets at reasonable prices. Lighter olive oils are also common now and less expensive still.

I was 12 when I first tasted olive oil. In the summer of 1954, lucky Family Ellis was on holiday in Lloret de Mar on the Costa Brava. It was Spanish olive oil that I sampled – an egg fried in this gorgeous green liquid. By golly it must have been good. I have been frying eggs in olive oil ever since.

Olive trees are ubiquitous in the Mediterranean region, where they grow in their millions. To see thousands of them en masse triggers the imagination and stays in the memory. On holiday in Corfu in the northeast of the island we saw a landscape thick with olive groves.

I remember standing in the arena at Delphi in 1961, the ancient olive groves, a shimmering carpet of grey–green sweeping down to the Gulf of Corinth.

When I told our friend Keith Richmond, who has an olive farm of a thousand trees southeast of Florence in the Tuscan hills, about this experience, he told me that in antiquity athletes used olive oil – I like to imagine from these same olive groves – to smear over their bodies at the Games in arenas like the one at Delphi. (Driving from the French border the 160km round the Ligurian coast to the Tuscan border, the terraced olive groves in November are covered in nets for the perilous business of harvesting.)

HERE ARE KEITH'S
CONTACT DETAILS:

Keith Richmond
Az. Agr. Boggioli
Loc. Boggioli, 10
52022 Montegonzi (AR), Italia
azienda@boggioli.com
www.boggioli.com

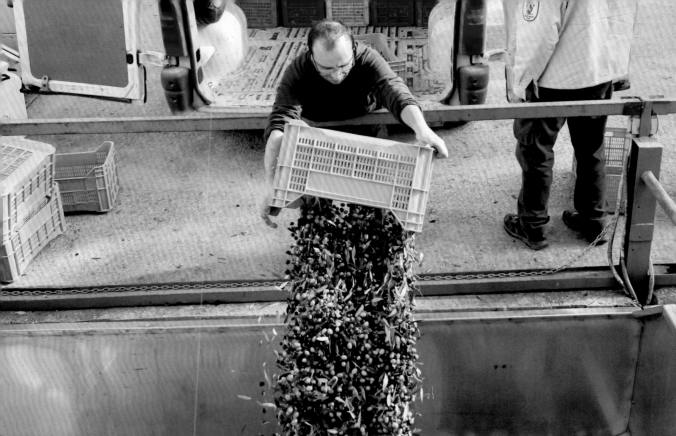

We empty the crates of olives into a huge steel funnel from where they make their way slowly into the processing plant. The days of large stone presses turned by donkeys are over …

In Andalusia in southern Spain, on the journey between Seville and Granada, olive plantations stretched 16km to the horizon.

On the isolated eastern fingertip of the Peloponnese on mainland Greece, I once saw a single olive tree, surrounded by a low, dry-stone wall. 'Keep out – family tree!' seemed to be the message.

It is seven in the morning and still dark as we bump over the rough-tracked shortcut from the farm, transporting the precious cargo of olives picked the day before to their fate. Keith and I are on our way to the local *frantoio* – where olives are transformed into oil. Keith says, 'Buy the best oil you can afford, organic if possible, and from somewhere you can trust.' He's a producer; he would say that, but I trust him and we have bought his oil for years. There is much chicanery in the olive industry, so it's best to know from whom you buy.

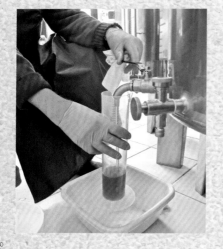

'As soon as you can, get them to the processor. They start degrading the moment they are picked. Two days maximum if you want to win any prizes.'

We are the first of the morning and avoid a long wait. We empty the crates of olives into a huge steel funnel from where they make their way slowly into the processing plant. The days of large stone presses turned by donkeys are over and now everything is done in a shiny steel centrifuge-based system of extraction. Even so, to see the first thin trickle of green gold emerge from the small tap at the end of the process is still a thrill.

We load the oil churns and take them back to the farm. On the table at lunch there is a small jug of this new, brilliant-green oil and we add it at will to our pasta and salad. Keith has a last piece of advice: to best preserve it keep it in a dark dispenser, glass or tin.

'And by golly it does you good.'

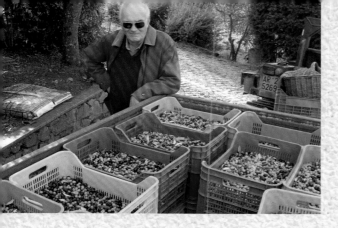

'Olive oil remains an essential part of everyday life and survival in this part of the world.'

Evidence from hundreds of studies, including Harvard Medical School, confirms its preventative and remedial powers. The list of benefits is impressive. Olive oil is rich in antioxidants, which fight against inflammation – a contributing cause of coronary artery disease, diabetes and other serious conditions. It follows that extra virgin olive oil can contribute to the body's fight against what Harvard Medical School describes as The Four Horsemen of the Medical Apocalypse: coronary artery disease, diabetes, cancer and Alzheimer's.

In the kitchen it is safe to use even at high temperatures. It is composed of 73% monounsaturated fat, 11% polyunsaturated fat and 14% saturated fat. The heat-resistant monounsaturated and saturated fats make up 87% of olive oil, thus countering the myth that it is unsuitable for frying. (See https://www.healthline.com)

It's common practice in restaurants everywhere now to offer as a pre-prandial treat what the Italians call *pinzimonio*, a saucer of quality extra virgin olive oil to dip your bread and raw vegetables into.

We've come a long way from the little bottles of 'medicinal' olive oil sold only in the chemists of my childhood – to put in your ear, not your mouth! Olive oil has become part of our daily lives – it's no longer necessary to go on holiday to the Costa Brava to taste an egg fried in olive oil. When it comes to olive oil, we are all Mediterraneans now.

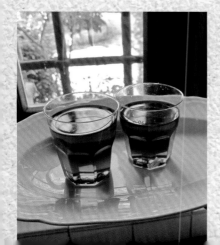

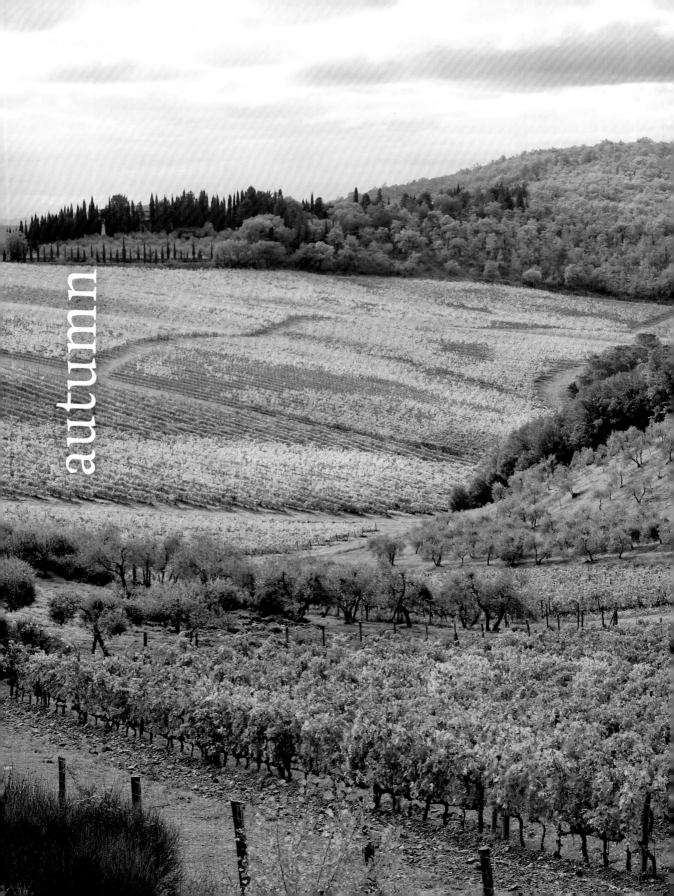

autumn

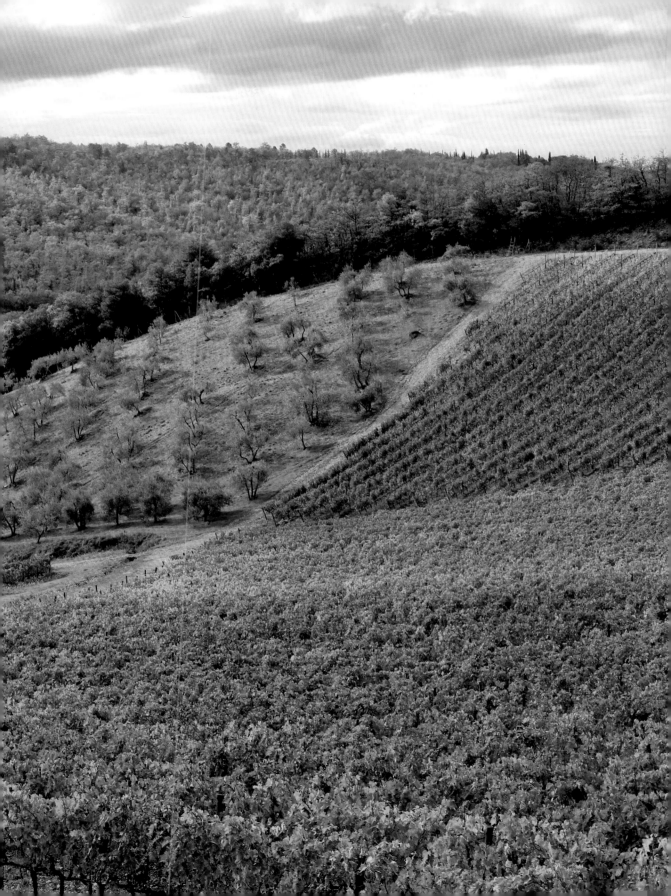

Autumn has everything. In culinary terms it is rich; the most diverse and varied of the seasons. The crown jewels of summer – tomatoes, aubergines, peppers, courgettes in mature splendour – still have two months in hand, offering mouth-watering opportunities and combinations.

And it is also the start of something. Buy a diary in France and you will notice that the year starts on September the first. In school terms it is called *la rentrée scolaire* – the re-start. The shop windows are full of satchels and writing materials. The rentrée is part of the cultural rhythm of France. The holidays are over and it's back to work we go.

The weeks pass into October and on to November. The colours change in the countryside around us and a refreshing sparseness emerges, as nature and the farmers get to work, clearing the old and preparing for the new. Starting over.

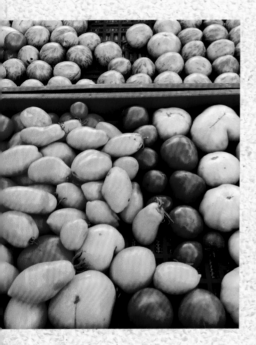

Harvests are gathered – sunflowers, wheat and barley – and celebrated, and by the end of November next year's garlic is planted for lifting in early July.

The market stalls are changing, too: the jewels are in retreat. Boxes of Roma tomatoes at attractive prices tempt us to search for those red rubber-seal preserving jars in the garage, give them a turn in the dishwasher and set them to work. It's not complicated and it's nice to have an alternative to a tin of tomatoes in winter.

The changes bring challenges and reminders and are welcome.

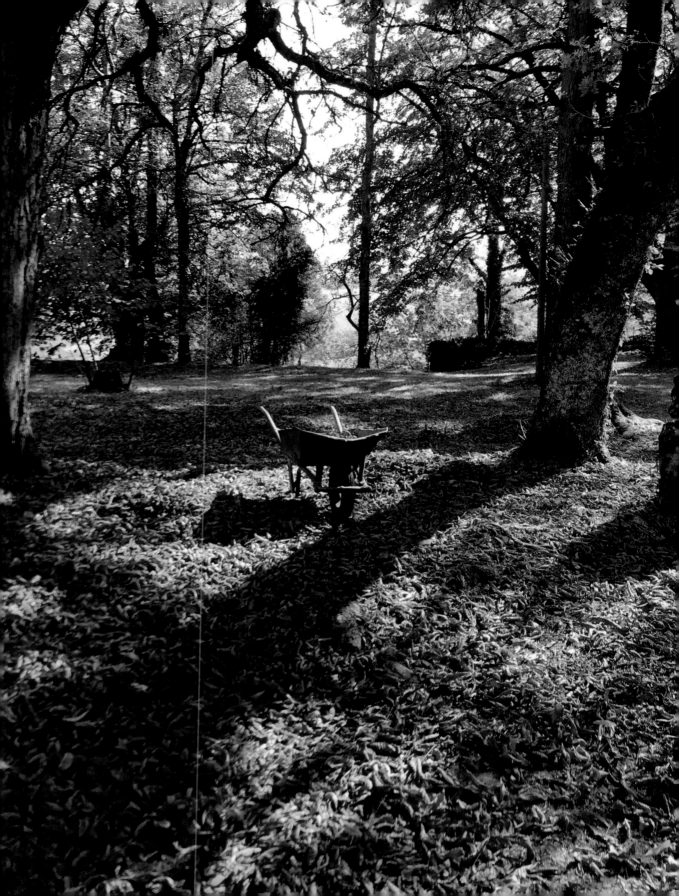

As the wind starts to bite, this gently warming soup eases us into autumn.

carrot, apple and ginger soup

SERVES 4

2 tbsp olive oil

1 onion, chopped

2 garlic cloves, crushed

2 tsp chopped ginger root

450g/1lb carrots, peeled and chopped, plus 1 whole carrot, peeled and halved

2 Fuji apples or apples of choice, peeled and chopped, plus 1 apple, finely diced

1 litre/4 cups vegetable stock

1 tsp salt

freshly ground black pepper

a few dashes of Tabasco (optional)

a bunch of chives, chopped, or a little flat-leaf parsley, to serve

1 Heat the olive oil in a large saucepan over medium heat. Add the onion, garlic and ginger and cook for about 3 minutes, until softened. Stir in the chopped carrots and apples (setting aside the diced apple), and cook for 1 minute, then add the halved carrot and the stock.

2 Bring the mixture to the boil, then reduce the heat and simmer, partly covered, for 30 minutes.

3 Remove the halved carrot using a slotted spoon. Chop it into fine dice and set aside.

4 Using a hand-held stick blender, blitz the soup until smooth.

5 Gently reheat the soup and season with the salt and a few grindings of pepper.

6 Serve the soup in bowls, garnished with the finely diced apples and carrots, a couple of shakes of Tabasco, if you wish, and a sprinkling of chopped chives or parsley.

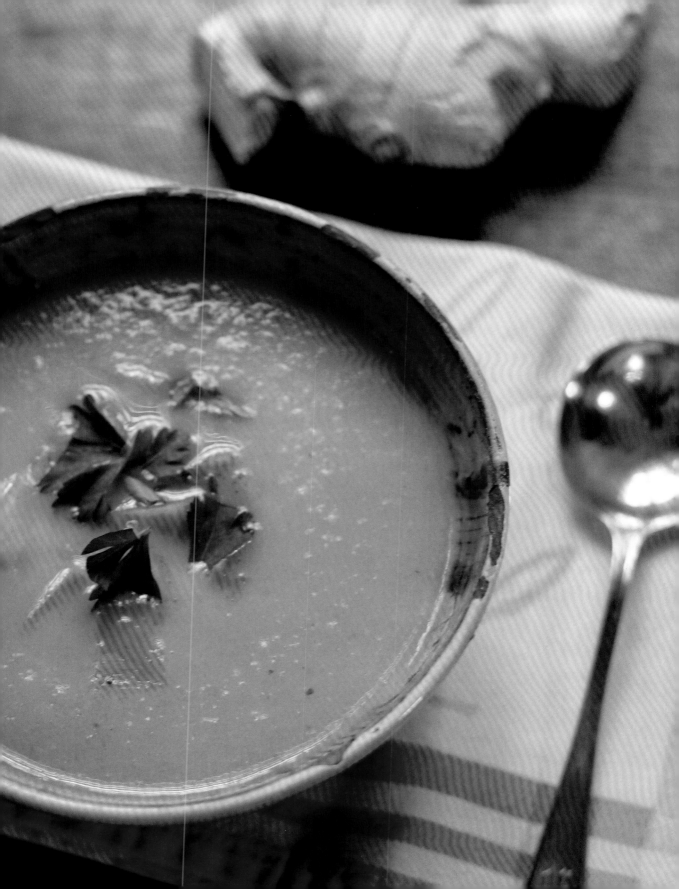

This is a soup for late-autumn evenings. Borlotti beans are the speckly ones – mottled white and red when uncooked. Cooking changes them to brown, which is a little disappointing. They have a nutty flavour that distinguishes them from cannellini beans and lends an air of gravity to this soup that white beans can't quite achieve. You can substitute white for borlotti, of course, if you prefer.

borlotti bean and cabbage soup

SERVES 4

1 tbsp olive oil, plus extra to serve

1 carrot, finely diced

1 onion, finely diced

1 celery stick, finely diced

1 garlic clove, chopped

1 tsp thyme leaves

400g/14oz tin of plum tomatoes, drained and chopped

400g/14oz tin of borlotti beans, drained

600ml/2½ cups vegetable stock

125g/4–5oz cabbage of choice (I use Savoy), finely chopped

salt and freshly ground black pepper

Parmesan cheese, grated, to serve

1 Heat the oil in a pan over a low heat. Add the carrot, onion, celery, garlic and thyme and cook gently for 7–8 minutes until softened.

2 Mix in the tomatoes, beans and stock, and season well with salt and plenty of freshly ground pepper to taste.

3 Bring the mixture up to a simmer, partly cover the pan and cook for 15 minutes. Stir in the cabbage and cook for a further 5 minutes until tender.

4 Serve hot with grated Parmesan and a swirl of olive oil. It tastes even better the day after…

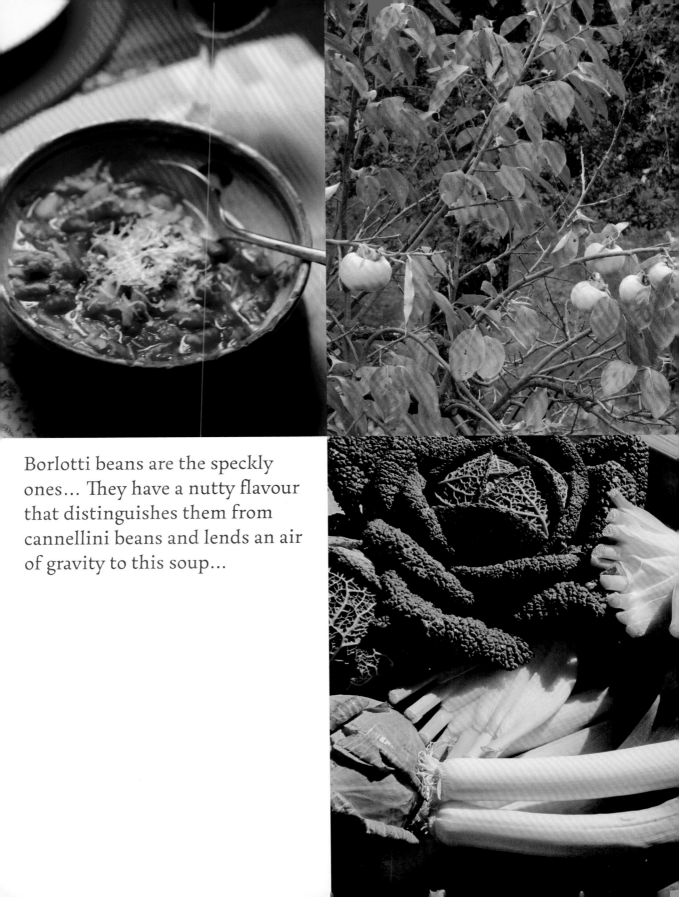

Borlotti beans are the speckly ones… They have a nutty flavour that distinguishes them from cannellini beans and lends an air of gravity to this soup…

I have happy memories of this Levantine salad. It is traditionally made with bulgur wheat, which here is replaced with hazelnuts. And I've added copious amounts of parsley. It featured as the starter on the first night of my cooking workshops. We'd all be a bit nervous settling in for the four days, not knowing one another. So lots of light chopping with an end in view gave us a focus. We'd set aside the ingredients and, just before sitting down to eat our first meal cooked as a team, we would build the tabbouleh in a large bowl, keeping the tomatoes until last to avoid a soggy starter.

roast hazelnut and parsley tabbouleh

SERVES 4–6 AS A STARTER

180g/6oz hazelnuts

2 bunches of flat-leaf parsley, lightly chopped

½ bunch fresh mint leaves, lightly chopped

1 large red onion, finely chopped

4 tomatoes, peeled, deseeded and diced

For the dressing

½ tsp allspice

⅓ tsp ground cinnamon

a good pinch of salt

juice of 2 lemons

1 tbsp hazelnut oil

6 tbsp olive oil

1 Preheat the oven to 180°C/350°F.

2 First, roast the hazelnuts. Scatter them over a baking tray and place in the oven for 10–12 minutes, until lightly coloured, taking care not to let them burn. Remove from the oven and allow to cool.

3 Meanwhile make the dressing by mixing together the allspice, cinnamon, salt and lemon juice in a bowl. Pour in the oils and mix thoroughly (or shake them together in a sealed jam jar). Set aside.

4 Shake the cooled nuts in a jar to remove as many brown skins as you can. Then whizz them in a food processor until crunchy (shingle not shale, i.e. not too fine).

5 Using your fingers and a light touch, carefully combine the herbs and the onion in a large serving bowl, then fold in the nuts. Add the diced tomatoes, pour over the dressing and mix tenderly to combine. The tabbouleh should look fresh, not soggy – although it'll taste good either way! Serve on a bed of mixed salad leaves or plain rocket.

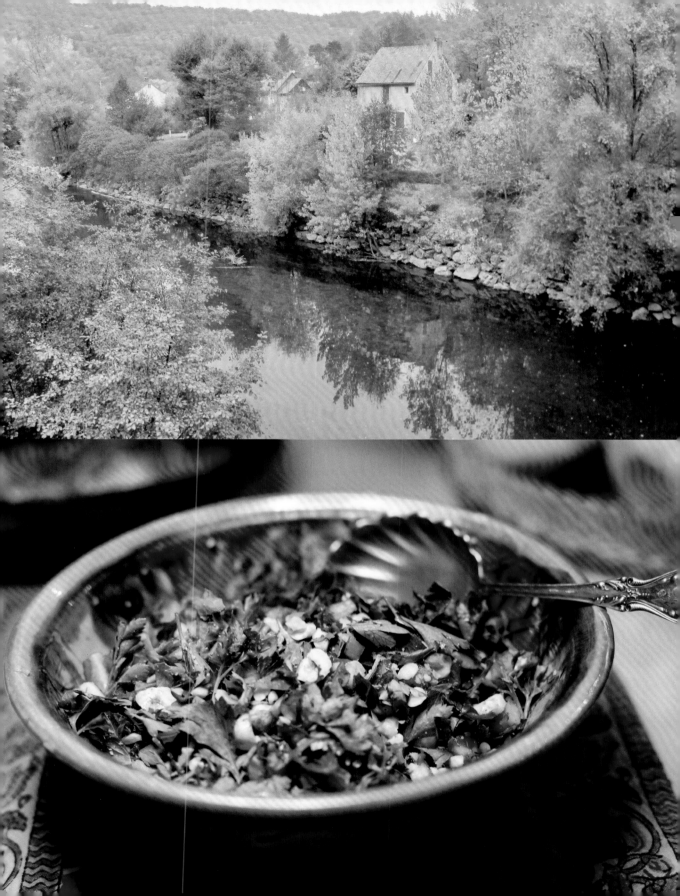

At the bar/restaurant San Niccolò in Radda in Chianti, the owner Caroline serves a traditional bruschetta, with fresh, brilliantly red-ripe diced tomatoes on slices of local bread. It's so good that after a bite of Meredith's, I have to order a plate, too.

White bread is not great for diabetics, so I've substituted a baked slice of aubergine – a tasty replacement. The trick is to spread the tomatoes just before serving; otherwise the slices become too soggy with the juice.

aubergine bruschetta

SERVES 4

1 tsp salt

2 large aubergines, peeled and sliced into thick rounds

2 tbsp olive oil, plus extra for brushing

red wine vinegar for brushing the aubergine slices after baking them

8 ripe tomatoes

2 garlic cloves, finely chopped, plus extra to taste, if necessary

2 basil leaves, snipped

freshly ground black pepper

1. Lightly salt the aubergine slices and leave them to drain in a colander for a couple of hours.

2. Preheat the oven to 220°C/425°F.

3. Wipe the aubergine slices dry with kitchen paper and brush both sides with olive oil. Lay them on an oiled baking tray and bake for 10 minutes on each side until nicely browned and soft. Remove from the oven, brush lightly with red wine vinegar and set aside.

4. Just before serving, prepare the tomatoes. Put them in a bowl and cover with boiling water. Leave for a minute. Fish them out and leave until cool enough to handle. Then remove the skins, halve, quarter and carefully deseed them. Then cut them into medium-sized dice.

5. Add the garlic, olive oil and basil and gently turn it all over – taking care not to make too much of a mush.

6. Spoon a generous amount of tomato mixture on to each aubergine slice and serve immediately.

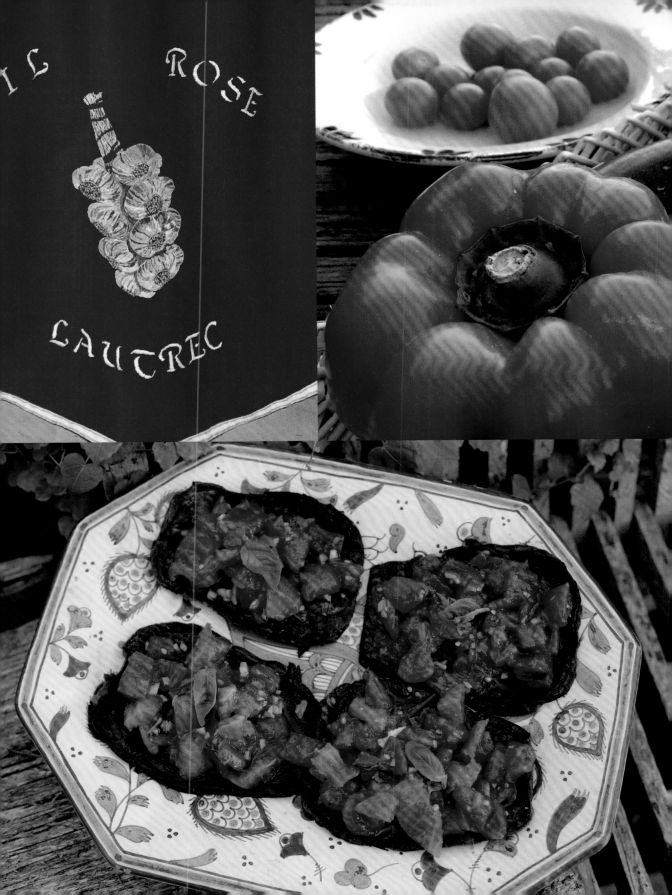

This is a useful variation on a favourite standby chez nous: stuffed peppers. I favour small red and yellow peppers for this. Two on a plate make a tasty starter, and they're nice to look at, too. Make four and you have a light lunch or supper. We love the creamy taste of emmental, but you could try substituting other cheeses, such as Parmesan, if you prefer. This is adapted from a Marcella Hazan recipe.

pepper boats with a light cargo

SERVES 2 OR 3

100g/3½oz small courgettes, sliced thinly in a food processor

50g/2oz emmental, grated

1 garlic clove, finely chopped

2 tbsp chopped flat-leaf parsley

25g/1oz organic wholegrain or rye breadcrumbs

3 tbsp olive oil, plus extra for brushing

3 smallish red peppers, peeled, deseeded and halved lengthways then halved again into cargo carrying, boat-shaped quarters

salt and freshly ground black pepper

1 Preheat the oven to 200°C/400°C.

2 In a large bowl mix the courgettes, cheese, garlic, parsley and breadcrumbs with 2 tablespoons of the olive oil. Season to taste.

3 Load the pepper boats generously with the courgette-mix cargo.

4 Line a baking tray with foil and brush with a little olive oil to 'moor' the boats ('How apt,' Meredith says. 'These boats being so "moreish"!') Sprinkle over the remaining tablespoon of olive oil and bake in the top half of the oven for 30 minutes or a little more if you think the peppers still need it.

5 Unload the sizzling boats onto plates and sail away.

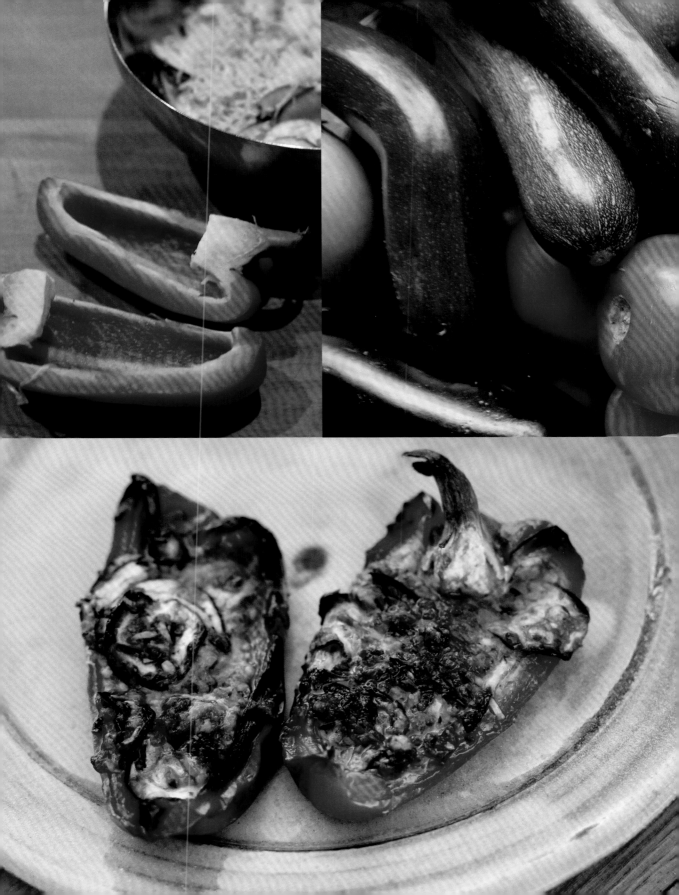

Autumn and mushrooms go together like a horse and carriage. As tomatoes take a bow until next year, mushrooms are popping up in forests and shops. This little dish serves nicely as a starter or even as a light lunch. As you delve deeper, it delivers layers of taste.

eggs en cocotte with mushrooms

SERVES 4

1 tbsp olive oil

250g/9oz mushrooms
(any type), quartered

zest of 1 lemon

a pinch of nutmeg

4 eggs

4 tsp crème fraîche

2 tbsp grated Parmesan

salt and freshly ground black pepper

1 Heat the oil in a shallow pan over a medium heat. Add the mushrooms and fry for a few minutes until they soften, lose their liquid and begin to take on some colour. Remove from the heat and set aside to cool.

2 While the mushrooms cool, combine the lemon zest and nutmeg on a small plate and season with salt and pepper. Scatter this over the mushrooms and mix lightly.

3 Lightly butter four ramekins.

4 Distribute the cooked mushrooms in the bottom of the ramekins. One at a time, break each egg into a small bowl, then slip it into a ramekin on top of the mushroom layer.

5 Add 1 teaspoon of crème fraîche into each ramekin and top each one with a quarter of the Parmesan.

6 Place a piece of kitchen paper in the bottom of a saucepan large enough to hold the four ramekins. (This is just to stop the rattling.) Carefully place the ramekins inside the pan and pour in enough boiling water to come three-quarters of the way up the outsides of the ramekins. It's important to avoid any water spilling into the ramekins.

7 Place the saucepan on a medium heat, bring the water back to a light boil and cover the pan for 3–4 minutes, then check to see if the eggs are done to your liking.

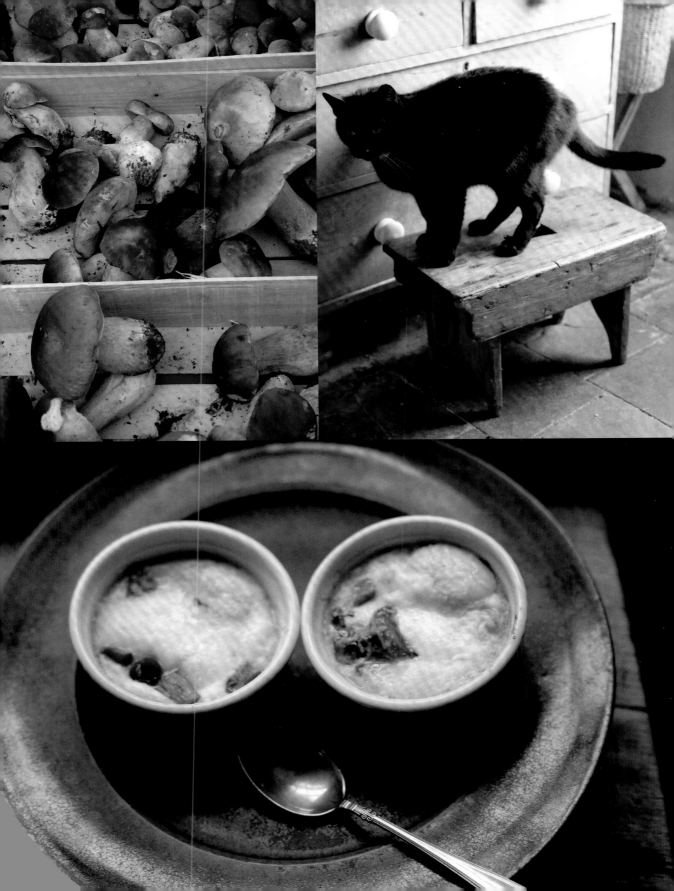

Our friend Romaine, a very good cook, introduced us to this easy-to-assemble, hard-to-stop-eating salad. It is a delicious mixture of soft white goat's cheese, diced beetroot and pan-roasted walnuts, served on young salad leaves with a balsamic dressing.

romaine's beetroot and goat's cheese salad

SERVES 4

4 handfuls of green salad leaves (such as lamb's lettuce, rocket and spinach)

6 spring onions, finely chopped

3 cooked beetroots, peeled and diced

a handful of lightly pan-roasted walnut kernels

1 small round of soft goat's cheese, roughly chopped

juice of ½ lemon, to serve

For the dressing

1 tbsp balsamic vinegar

1 tsp Dijon mustard

3 tbsp olive oil

salt and freshly ground black pepper

1 Lay out the salad leaves on a shallow salad dish. Top with the spring onions, then the beetroot, walnut kernels and chopped goat's cheese.

2 Combine the dressing ingredients in a small bowl or lidded jam jar and season with salt and pepper.

3 Pour the dressing over the salad and turn carefully to mix everything together.

4 To serve, sprinkle over the lemon juice.

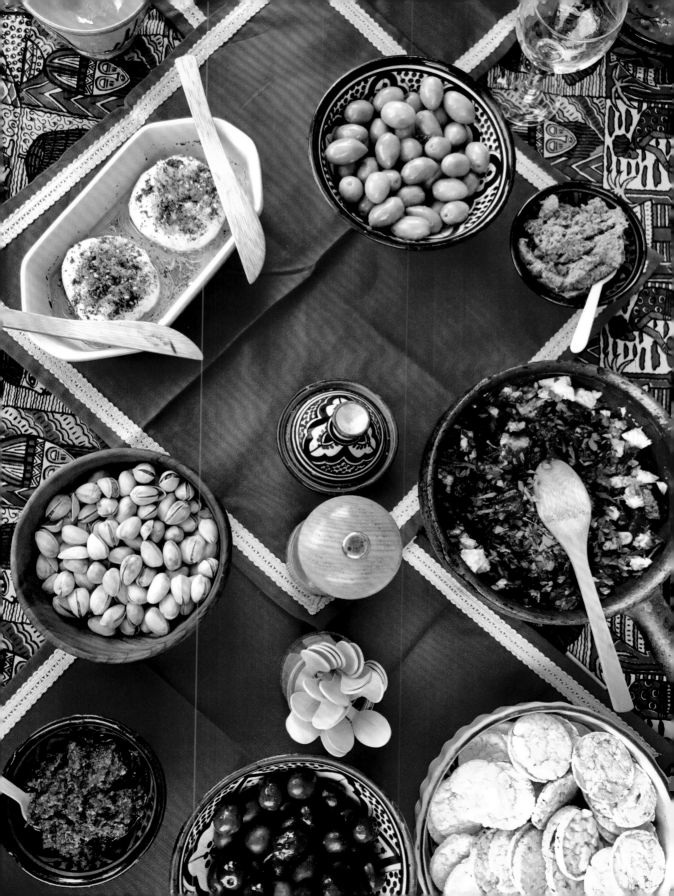

This is a mezze-like, serve-yourself starter. There are, as with many North African dishes, a multitude of versions and several names, all of them on the theme of peppers and spices. FELFLA – I like the name. Add an A, rearrange the letters and you have FALAFEL – the chickpea wonder. Chickpeas feature in this, too, mixed in with soft goat's cheese and a garlicky lemon dressing.

felfla

SERVES 4

3 tbsp olive oil, plus extra for brushing

4 large red peppers, or a mixture of yellow and red

1 large garlic clove, pulped in a mortar with a pinch of salt

1 tbsp lemon juice

400g/14oz tin of chickpeas, drained

1 tsp ground cumin

1 small soft goat's cheese, roughly chopped

salt and freshly ground black pepper

1 Preheat the oven to 200°C/400°F.

2 Cover a shallow baking tray with a sheet of foil and brush lightly with oil. Add the peppers and place in the upper part of the oven to roast for about 40 minutes, turning a couple of times during cooking, until they are nicely charred. Remove from the oven and leave in the tray to cool.

3 Make a dressing. Put the garlic, lemon juice and olive oil in a small bowl, season with salt and pepper, and stir well to combine (or put in a jam jar, replace the lid and shake it all about to combine).

4 Put the chickpeas in a bowl. Sprinkle over the cumin and stir to combine. Lay the goat's cheese on the chickpeas and add a spoonful of the dressing – it will benefit from a few minutes marinating.

5 Peel the cooled peppers and deseed them.

6 You are now ready to assemble the salad. Choose a shallow serving dish and lay out the pepper flesh in a pretty fashion in the dish. Spoon over 2 tablespoons of the dressing and give the dish a little shake to distribute the dressing. Carefully spoon over the chickpea and goat's cheese mixture, to serve.

This is a useful recipe for end-of-season French beans – you can never have too many ideas for cooking green beans. Here, they are bathed in a little lemony cheese sauce to serve as a starter or as a salad or even as a side vegetable to a main dish.

green beans with parmesan

SERVES 4

2 tsp salt

450g/1lb green beans, topped

zest of 1 lemon and 2 tbsp juice

6 tbsp olive oil

50g/2oz Parmesan, grated

1 Bring a saucepan of water to the boil. Add the salt and the beans, and bring back to the boil.

2 Test for doneness after 5 minutes. The beans should be tender but do not overcook.

3 Whisk together the lemon juice, zest and oil in a large bowl. Gradually whisk in the cheese to form a sauce.

4 Drain the beans and transfer them to the bowl with the sauce, turning to coat. Serve at once or tepid as a salad.

5 If you prefer, you could roast the beans to almost done, then add a sprinkling of Parmesan before popping them back in the oven for a final 10 minutes – as with the roasted asparagus recipe (see p.31) in the Spring section.

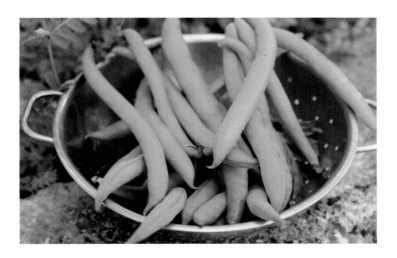

Years ago, we had lunch at a traditional brasserie in Toulouse and I chose as a starter a salad that sounded a little different. It was an assembly of baby gem lettuce (called sucrine *here, as they have a sweetness to them), small dollops of tapenade, Parmesan shavings and quails' eggs. It looked beautiful: green and black with the yellow of the egg yolks and Parmesan. It tasted good, too – and joined my repertoire of starters.*

This version takes that recipe further, adding the smoky edge that grilling gives the lettuce halves. These tightly formed little gems keep their shape and are transformed into main players on the plate.

grilled baby gem with egg topping

SERVES 4

4 baby gem or small romaine lettuce hearts, halved lengthways

4 tbsp Tapenade (see p.212) or chopped black olives

a pinch of Parmesan shavings, to serve

4 poached eggs

For the dressing

6 tbsp olive oil, plus extra for brushing

2 tbsp red wine vinegar

salt and freshly ground black pepper

1 First, combine the ingredients for the dressing in a small bowl.

2 Heat a griddle pan to hot.

3 Brush the cut side of the lettuce halves with the dressing and a little more olive oil.

4 Grill one side while lightly brushing the other sides with the dressing. The grilling should take long enough to soften and char the lettuce without burning – about 3–4 minutes for the first side.

5 Carefully turn over the lettuce halves and grill for a further 2 minutes or so, until both sides are nicely softened and charred.

6 Place two lettuce halves on each plate and spoon a little more dressing over each (keep any leftover dressing for another time). Top with dollops of tapenade or juicy black olives and some Parmesan shavings and finish with the poached eggs.

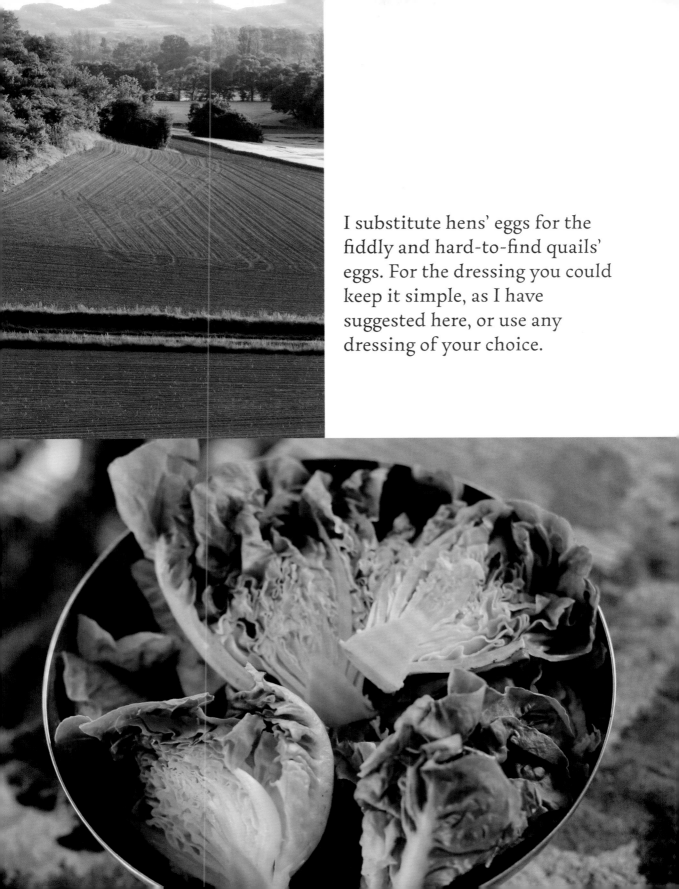

I substitute hens' eggs for the fiddly and hard-to-find quails' eggs. For the dressing you could keep it simple, as I have suggested here, or use any dressing of your choice.

The ideal time for this dish is late summer and early autumn. Aubergines are in their pomp, peppers are plump and sweet and tomatoes are effortlessly delicious. I made it the other night just for the two of us – it was oily and unctuous. The trick here is separate pans and patience.

autumn ratatouille

SERVES 2 OR 3

1 large aubergine

·1 large courgette

6 tbsp olive oil, plus extra if needed

1 red pepper, peeled, deseeded and cut into squares

1 medium onion, chopped

2 garlic cloves, pulped with a pinch of salt

2 tomatoes, peeled, deseeded and chopped

pinch of dried oregano

salt and freshly ground black pepper

1 Peel the aubergine and courgette to create stripes: using a hand peeler, peel a 5cm strip, leave a 5cm gap and then peel again. Cut into 2cm/¾in dice, then place them into separate sieves, sprinkle with salt and leave to drain into separate bowls for 1 hour. Remove from the sieves and squeeze the remaining liquid out of them using kitchen paper.

2 Fry them in separate pans on a medium to low heat in 2 tablespoons of olive oil for each pan, turning them as they brown and become completely soft. This is where patience joins the list of ingredients! You may need to add a little more oil to the aubergine pan.

3 Turn off the heat and empty one pan into the other. Heat a further 2 tablespoons of oil in the empty pan. Add the pepper squares and onion and cook on a medium heat for 10 minutes, until browned and soft. Stir in the garlic, allowing it to soften but not brown for a couple of minutes, then add the tomatoes and oregano. Mix well.

4 Cook for 5 minutes to let the tomatoes break down, then add this mixture to the pan with the aubergines and courgettes, along with 4 tablespoons of water. Stir to mix. Cook over a low heat for 15 minutes to allow 'unctuousness' to happen – don't rush it and be careful it doesn't burn.

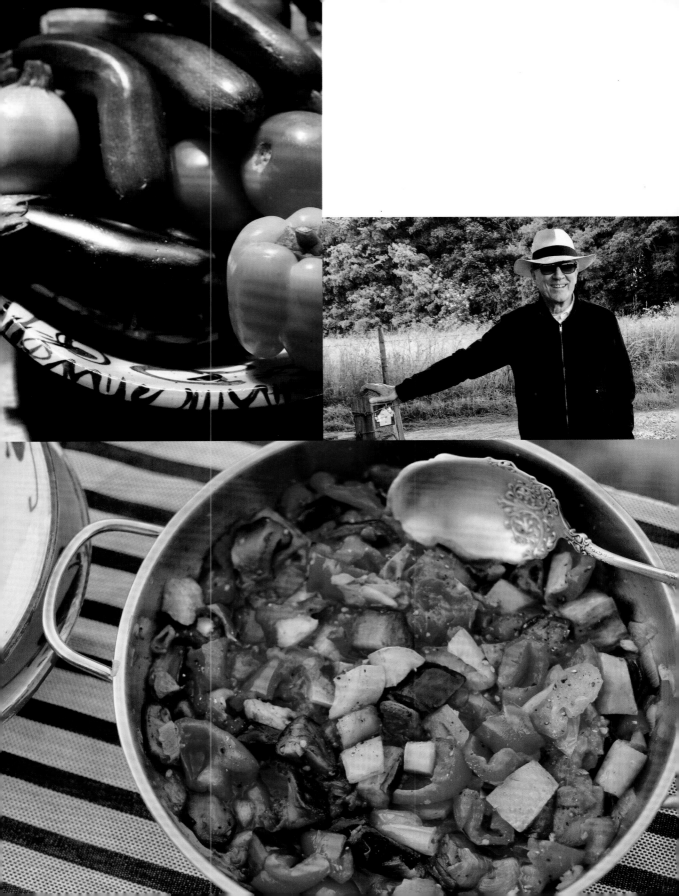

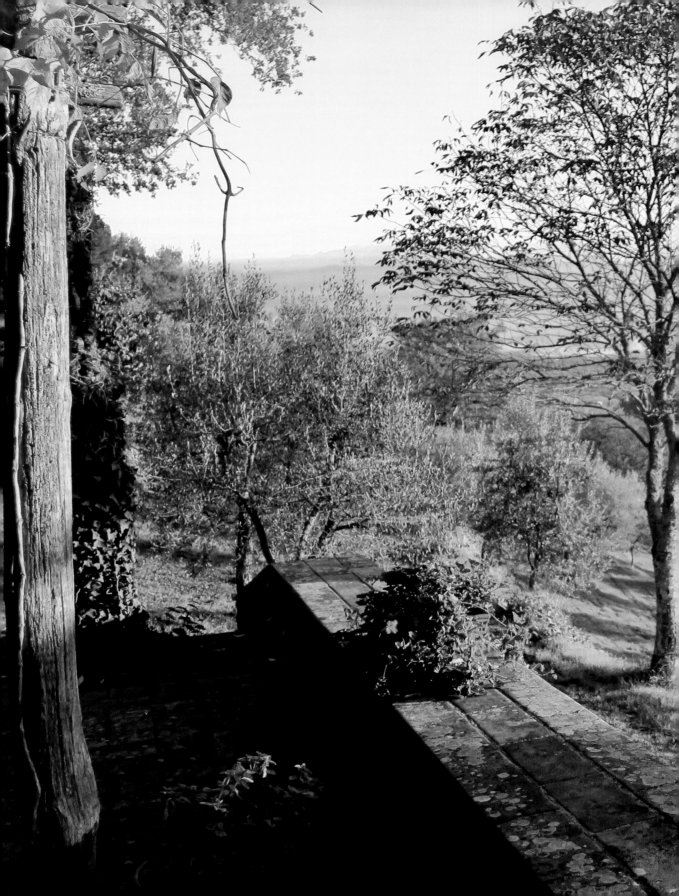

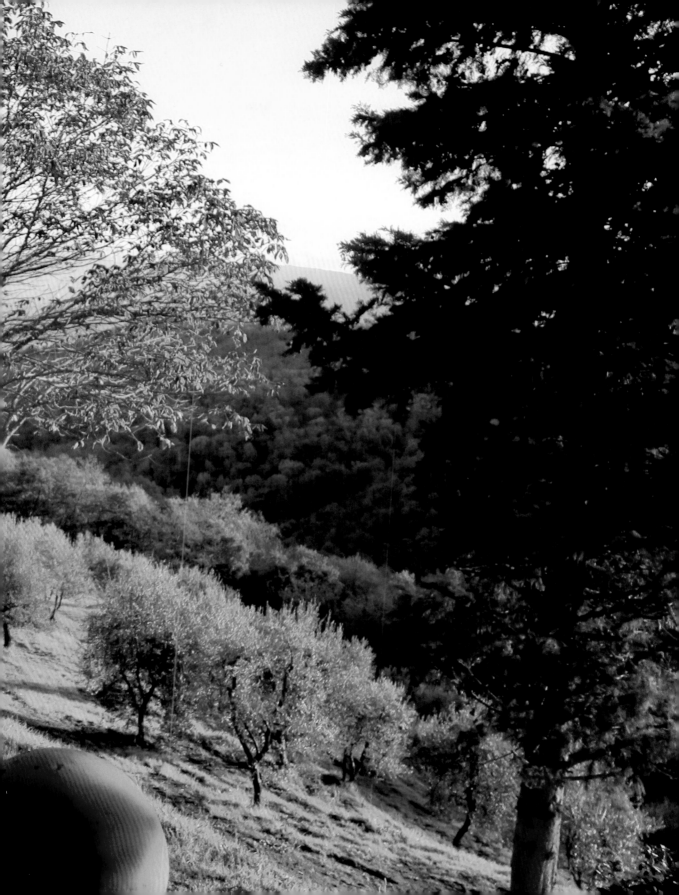

Our neighbour Flo left us eggs and onions in exchange for feeding her cats and hens while she and her husband spent a few well-earned days' rest in Corsica. Not strictly Mediterranean, this lovely mess of eggs in an onion, red pepper and tomato sauce is from the Basque Country that borders the Atlantic Ocean in southwest France and northwest Spain. The name comes from the Latin for pepper, piperis. Red peppers, onions and tomatoes are softened into a sauce and given a subtle kick by the local, mildly spicy piment d'Espelette – although a pinch of cayenne will do the job. Beaten eggs are then scrambled into the mixture to finish.

piperade

SERVES 3 OR 4

2 tbsp olive oil

400g/14oz onions, sliced or chopped

1 garlic clove, crushed with a pinch of salt

3 red peppers, peeled (see p.82), deseeded and sliced into strips

400g/14oz tomatoes, skinned and roughly chopped; or 400g tin of tomatoes, drained and chopped

1 bay leaf

a sprig of thyme

1 tsp *piment d'Espelette* or ⅓ tsp cayenne pepper

6 eggs, beaten

salt and freshly ground black pepper

1   Heat the oil in a medium saucepan over a low heat. Add the onions and garlic and cook for 20 minutes, until soft. Add the peppers and turn to combine, then cover the pan and cook for about 10 minutes, to soften them.

2   Add the tomatoes, herbs and spice, stir to combine and then season with salt and pepper. Cook covered for 10 minutes, then remove the lid and cook for a further 10 minutes to steam off some of the excess liquid.

3   Add the beaten eggs to the sauce and turn over gently, until the eggs are done as you like them. Serve immediately.

Traditionally, the dish would be served with a locally cured ham – but not in this book! I serve it with a green salad. Comfort food and lunch today as summer leans into autumn.

This recipe is adapted from a dish in Margot Henderson's book You're All Invited.

braised fennel with green olives and orange peel

SERVES 2 (GENEROUSLY)

3 tbsp olive oil

3 large fennel bulbs, trimmed, cut into 1cm/½in wedges and halved again

5 garlic cloves, peeled

strips of peel from 1 orange

2 strips of lemon peel

large glass of white wine

a sprig of thyme and 3 bay leaves, tied together with string

12 green olives, pitted

salt and freshly ground black pepper

1 Preheat the oven to 180°C/350°F.

2 Heat the oil in an ovenproof pan over a medium heat and add the fennel. Sauté for 15 minutes or until lightly browned.

3 Add the garlic cloves and both peels. Cook for 2–3 minutes, then add the wine, herbs and olives. Season to taste with salt and pepper. Gently bring to the boil and simmer for a couple of minutes to allow the ingredients to get to know each other. Cover the pan and cook in the oven for 45 minutes – the fennel must be tender – (check after 30 minutes, if you like).

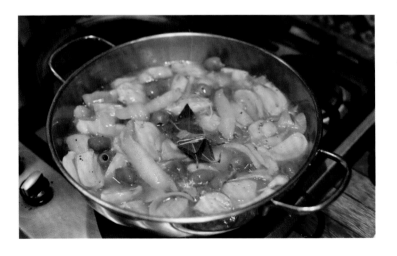

Something to do on a slow day! Patience is ever the extra ingredient that makes the difference between dry and moist frittatas. In this case, patience to melt the sliced onion slowly and not to rush the cooking of the egg mixture. Choose a 26cm/10½in frying pan with a heatproof handle that fits under the grill, to make the frittata.

red onion frittata

SERVES 3 OR 4

6 tbsp olive oil

450g/1lb red onions, thinly sliced

5 eggs

50g/2oz Parmesan, grated

salt and freshly ground black pepper

1 Heat the oil in a large frying pan over a low heat. Add the onions and sauté for about 20 minutes, or until they start to caramelise and that pleasing scent wafts over the kitchen.

2 Turn off the heat and prop up the pan at an angle to allow some of the oil to drain to one side and the onions to cool, then spoon out the drained oil into the 26cm/10½in frying pan. You'll need 2 tablespoons – so top up with extra olive oil if necessary. Set aside.

3 Beat the eggs in a bowl. Add the onions and the Parmesan to the beaten eggs and season well with salt and pepper.

4 Heat the oil in the pan until hot. Add the egg mixture and spread evenly to cover the base. Turn the heat to its lowest setting and cook the frittata for about 30 minutes (a heat diffuser is useful for keeping the heat even and low).

5 Meanwhile, heat the grill to hot.

6 When there is just a pool of loose egg mix left on top, place the pan under the grill for about 1 minute, until the top is lightly coloured. Ease a spatula under and around the frittata and slide it on to a serving plate.

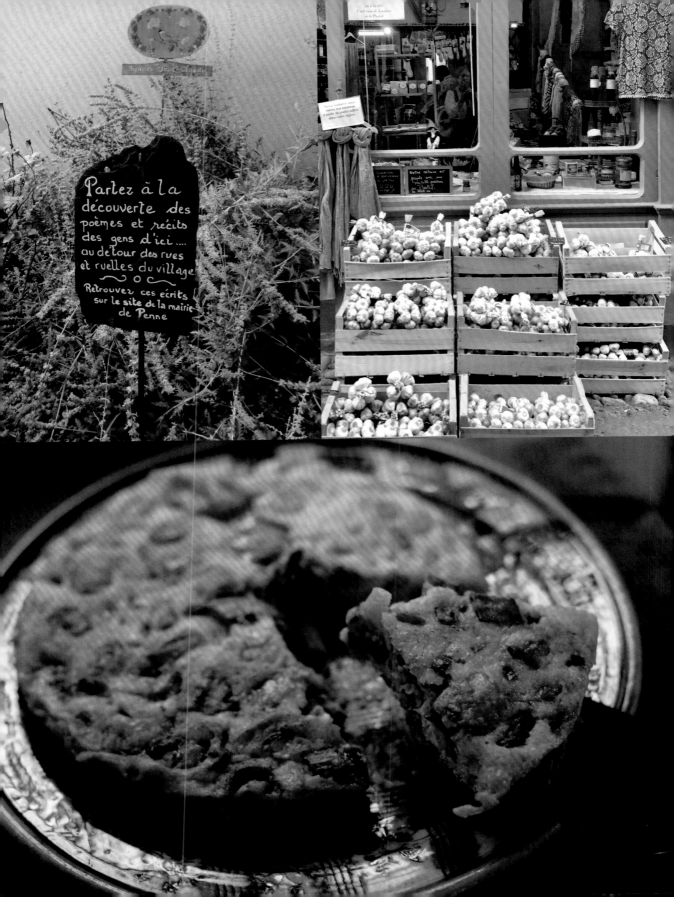

Partez à la
découverte des
poèmes et récits
des gens d'ici....
au détour des rues
et ruelles du village
○
Retrouvez ces écrits
sur le site de la mairie
de Penne

In truth there isn't much of the Mediterranean about this dish; it's more typical of inland cuisine. It's useful, though, when the courgettes are piling up in the crisper. To give it a 'view of the Med' serve with Red Pepper Boats (p.124) or a ripe tomato salad. Adapted from a recipe in the wonderful Jenny Baker's Simple French Cuisine.

courgette gratin

SERVES 2 OR 3

1 tbsp olive oil

700g/1½lb courgettes, thinly sliced in a food processor

a sprig of rosemary

1 egg

4 tbsp ricotta

a pinch of nutmeg – easy with the nutmeg!

2–3 tbsp or more grated emmental or Parmesan

salt and freshly ground black pepper

1 Preheat the oven to 200°C/400°F.

2 Heat the oil in a medium pan. Add the courgettes and rosemary sprig, then turn the heat to low and cover the pan. Cook for about 15 minutes, until the courgettes are very tender.

3 Meanwhile, break the egg into a bowl. Add the ricotta and the pinch of nutmeg, season with salt and pepper and mix thoroughly. Taste, and adjust the seasoning if necessary.

4 Remove the cooked courgettes from the heat, allow to cool a little, then tip them into the bowl with the ricotta mixture and mix until nicely coated.

5 Transfer the mixture to a medium terracotta gratin dish, scatter over the cheese and bake in the upper part of the oven for about 30 minutes until nicely browned on top.

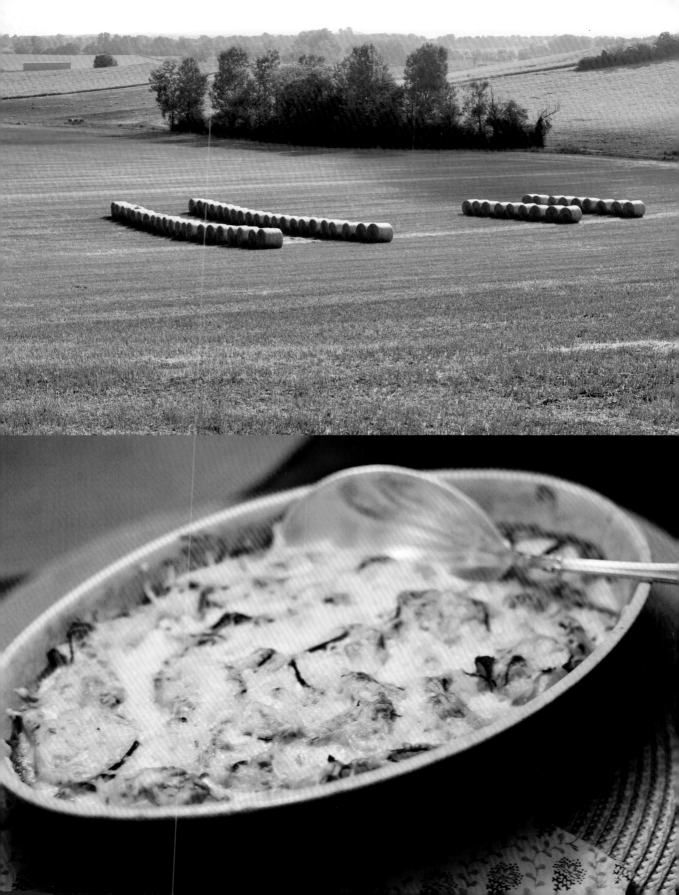

This delicious dish of chickpeas, cumin and lemon is very quick and very simple, making it perfect for when you have company. I have adapted it from a recipe in a delightful book called Recipes from Home, a collection of Syrian recipes from women separated from their homeland by the war in their country and collated by Itam Azzam and Dina Mousami.

Balihla has versions in the cuisines of every country, every region and every household bordering the middle eastern and north African Mediterranean. The common factors are chickpeas, cumin and lemon.

balihla

SERVES 4

400g/14oz tin of chickpeas

1 medium tomato, diced

1 garlic clove, finely chopped

1 tsp salt, plus extra to taste

juice of 1 lemon, plus extra to taste

4 tbsp olive oil, plus extra to taste

2 tsp ground cumin

2 tbsp finely chopped flat-leaf parsley

a good handful of salad leaves, to serve

a bunch of spring onions, sliced

1 Gently heat the chickpeas with their liquid in a shallow pan. When warmed through, pour them into a serving bowl, ditching some of the liquid, and mix in the diced tomato.

2 Whisk the garlic, salt, lemon juice and olive oil together into a sauce, pour three tablespoons over the chickpeas and mix it in.

3 Sprinkle over the cumin and check the seasoning, then scatter the spring onions and parsley over the top. Serve on a bed of salad leaves.

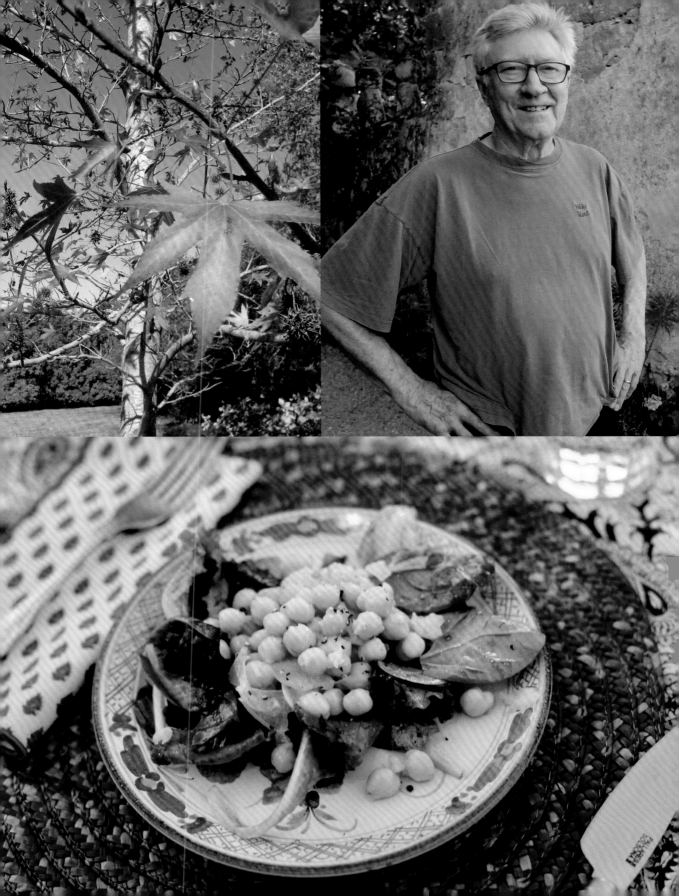

A nifty lunch, this – with, if you fancy, a poached egg on top. Cooking the beans longer may be anathema to some but give it a try; you may find it hard to leave any leftovers!

greek green beans with tomato, cumin and feta

SERVES 2 OR 3

4 tbsp olive oil

1 onion, roughly chopped

2 garlic cloves, chopped

450g/1lb ripe tomatoes, skinned, deseeded and roughly chopped

1 tsp ground cumin

1 thyme sprig

1 bay leaf

¼ tsp cayenne, or ½ small red chilli, chopped

250g/9oz green beans, halved

salt and freshly ground black pepper

100g/3½oz feta cheese or more, crumbled, to serve

lightly poached eggs (optional), to serve

1 Heat 3 tablespoons of the olive oil in a medium saucepan over a medium heat. Reduce the heat to low and add the onion. Cook for 2–3 minutes, turning in the oil, then add the garlic. Cook for a further 10 minutes or until the onion has softened nicely. Then add half the tomatoes with the cumin, thyme, bay and cayenne or chilli, and season lightly with salt and pepper.

2 Lay the beans over the top to cover the tomato mixture. Then cover the beans with the remaining tomatoes and season lightly again. Sprinkle over the remaining tablespoon of olive oil. Cover the pan and increase the heat to bring up to the boil.

3 As soon as the mixture starts to boil, reduce the heat to low again and cook, covered, for 20 minutes, then remove the lid and cook for a further 20 minutes.

4 To serve sprinkle on the feta and add a lightly poached egg on top, if that suits.

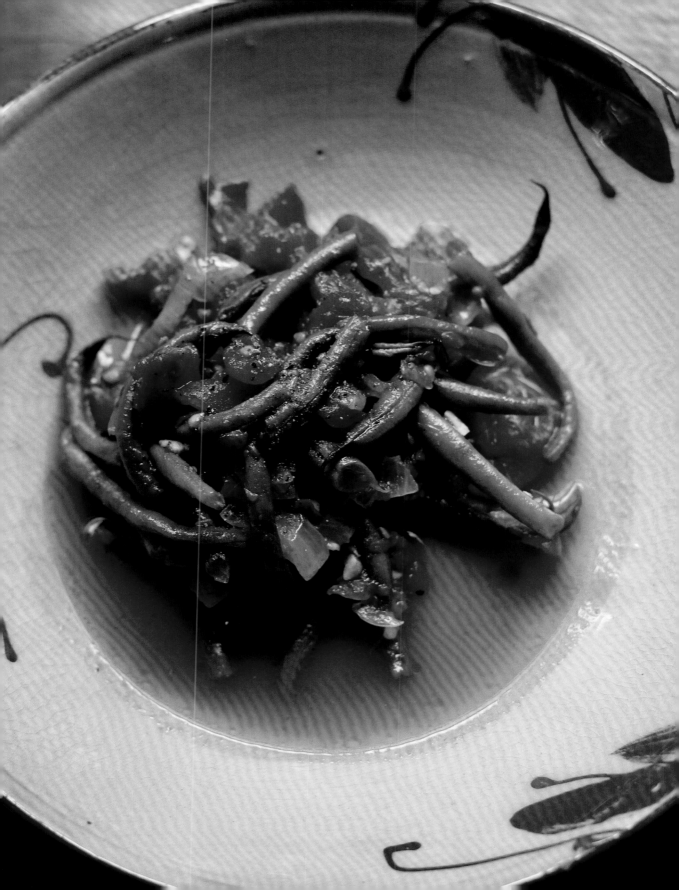

This dish is soft and comforting and a good background to a light autumn supper. Late green beans or early broccoli would complement, with new garlic and olive oil adding a little kick. Meredith, a lentil sceptic on account of their reputation for windiness, couldn't help helping herself to more!

curried green lentils for a changing season

SERVES 3 OR 4

3 tbsp olive oil

1 onion, chopped

3 tsp madras curry powder or curry powder of choice

3 tbsp tomato concentrate

1 tsp salt

200g/generous 1 cup green lentils

750ml/3 cups vegetable stock

sweet onion slices (optional, but delicious), for sprinkling

1 Heat the oil in a medium saucepan, add the onion and gently soften for 6–7 minutes.

2 Add the curry powder, tomato concentrate, salt and lentils, and stir well together, adding a couple of tablespoons of the stock to loosen it all. Stir in the rest of the stock and cover the pan. Let it cook on a low heat for 30 minutes – stirring from time to time, until the lentils are cooked through and tender (cook for a little while longer, if they aren't).

3 Serve in bowls, sprinkled with chopped onion if you wish.

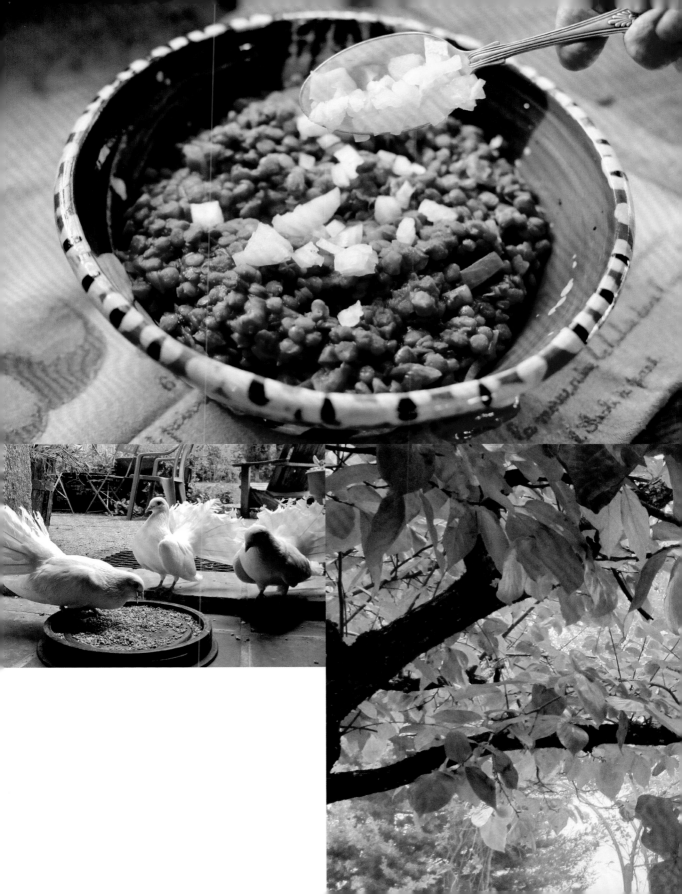

A consoling casserole for a cold autumn night, this dish is inspired by a recipe in the River Café Pocket Vegetable Book. I love beans, especially white beans, and I have a penchant for fennel, cooked or raw. Garlic is a staple where we live – Lautrec's pink garlic is grown under our feet, so to speak. Adding tomatoes coalesces everything into a delicious dish.

fennel, tomatoes and white beans

SERVES 2 (JUST!)

2 tbsp olive oil

2 fennel bulbs, outer bruised parts removed and cut in thick vertical slices

3 garlic cloves, sliced

1 tsp fennel seeds, pounded in a mortar

2 small dried chillies, chopped

250g/9oz tinned tomatoes, drained and chopped

400g/14oz of white beans, drained

juice of 1 lemon

salt and freshly ground black pepper

1 Heat 1 tablespoon of the olive oil in a shallow pan over a medium heat. Add the fennel and cook for 2–3 minutes, turning the fennel over in the oil. Add the garlic, fennel seeds and chillies and cook for 5 minutes, then add the tomatoes. Stir to combine, then add 1 tablespoon of water and stir again. Cover the pan and cook for about 15 minutes, or until the fennel is tender. (Check the sauce after 5 minutes and add another 1 tablespoon of water to loosen the sauce a little if you need to – I did.)

2 Remove the lid and stir in the beans. Season with salt and pepper, then replace the lid and cook for a further 10 minutes. Add the lemon juice and the second tablespoon of olive oil.

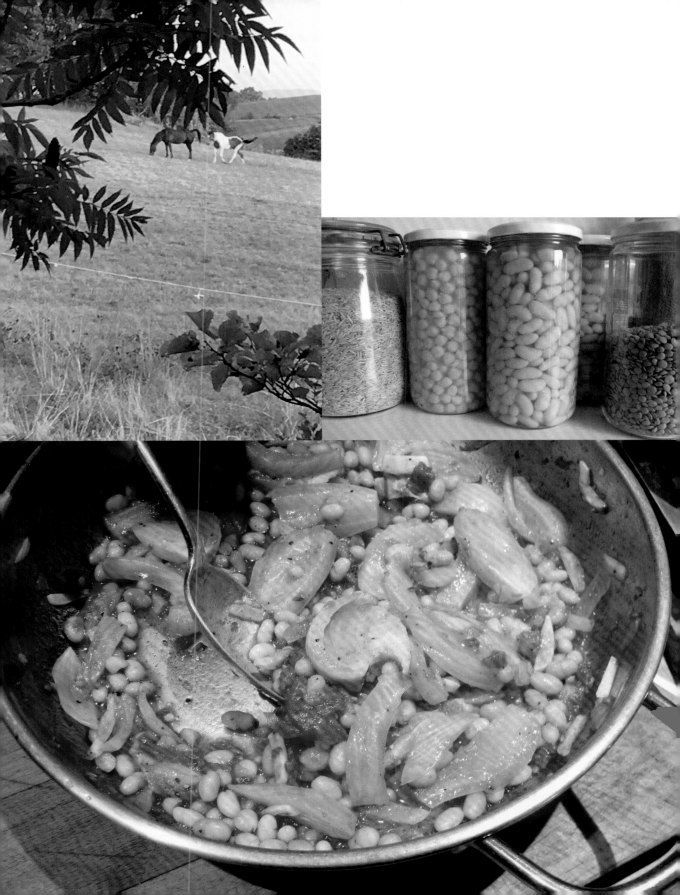

A subtly flavoured dish from the eastern Mediterranean, sometimes combining rice with the lentils and sometimes, as here, bulgur wheat. Slowly caramelised onions are added to the cooked bulgur and lentils and then an encore of faster cooked crispy onions spread on top. It's easy to make and useful as a side dish or the main player.

mujadara (spicy lentils and bulgur wheat with onions)

SERVES 4

2 tbsp olive oil

2 large onions, roughly chopped

1 tsp ground cumin

1 tsp ground coriander

½ tsp allspice

¼ cayenne pepper

200g/7oz puy or brown lentils

100g/3½oz bulgur wheat

½ tsp salt

For the crispy onions

3 tbsp olive oil for frying

2 onions, thinly sliced

1 Heat the olive oil in a large frying pan and when it is hot put in the onions. Let these brown nicely on a medium–low heat for about 40 minutes while you are cooking the lentils and bulgur.

2 Put 500ml/2 cups of water in a medium saucepan and add the cumin, coriander, allspice and cayenne.

3 Add the lentils and bring up to the simmer. Cover and cook for 20 minutes or until the lentils are almost cooked (retaining a little bite). Add the bulgur wheat (there should be enough water left but add a little extra water if needed) and the salt.

4 Cover again and cook for a further 10 minutes until the bulgur wheat is soft. Then turn off the heat and leave aside, covered.

5 When the onions are caramelised, drain the oil into a bowl and mix the onions into the lentils.

6 To make the crispy onions, heat the reserved oil and the 3 tablespoons of olive oil in the frying pan; add the thinly sliced onions and cook them on a medium–high heat, stirring often, for about 10 minutes, until they become golden and crispy, taking care not to burn them.

7 Remove them from the oil.

8 Spoon the lentil and bulgur mixture on to a serving plate and pile the crispy onions on top.

Chard is bulky and a touch intimidating: flappy leaves attached to hard white or coloured stalks.
I bought a kilo in the market this morning – it's a job fitting a kilo of it into a paper bag. It can look
a bit droopy, too, so the fresher the better; this batch was shining with freshness.

spicy swiss chard

SERVES 4

1kg/2lb 4oz Swiss chard, leaves and stalks separated

1 tsp salt

4 garlic cloves, 1 left whole, 3 sliced

3 tbsp olive oil

1 dried chilli, chopped with seeds

1   Pile the chard leaves together – or make two piles, if necessary – and slice across in two or three places. Turn the piles through 180° and repeat so that you end up with rough squares.

2   Slice the chard stems into roughly 2.5cm/1in dice.

3   Bring a large saucepan of water to the boil over a high heat. Add the salt and the chard leaves. Cover and bring back to the boil. Test the leaves after 2–3 minutes – they are cooked when they melt in the mouth.

4   Using a slotted spoon, lift out the leaves into a colander (leave the water on the boil) and let them cool before squeezing out the excess water (take care not to burn yourself). Set aside.

5   Put the whole garlic clove into the boiling water. Add the chopped chard stems and cook for about 5 minutes, or until tender. Drain and set aside.

6   Gently heat the olive oil in a pan large enough to take both the leaves and stems. Add the sliced garlic. When it starts to colour after a few minutes, add the chilli and, after a brief pause, the chard leaves and stems. Turn it all over in the garlicky oil for a couple of minutes to warm through, then serve immediately.

Gratins are so handy and work equally well either as accompanying dishes or as the main event. The rosemary, garlic and chilli flakes here enhance the sweet aniseed flavour of the fennel. This is quick to assemble and, of course, delicious. Pecorino is ewe's cheese with a light saltiness to it; if you prefer, you can just use double the amount of Parmesan.

two-cheese fennel gratin

SERVES 3 OR 4

4 large fennel bulbs, tough outer layers removed, sliced to give 4 or 5 slices per bulb

1 tsp fennel seeds

3 tbsp olive oil

a pinch of chilli flakes

2 garlic cloves, crushed with a pinch of salt

1 tsp very finely chopped rosemary needles

50g/2oz Parmesan, grated

50g/2oz wholegrain or rye breadcrumbs

50g/2oz pecorino Romano, grated

salt and freshly ground black pepper

1 Place the fennel slices in a steamer (or in a colander over a pan of boiling water) and cook until tender. While the fennel is steaming, lightly toast the fennel seeds in a dry frying pan and set aside.

2 In a bowl, mix together the fennel seeds, olive oil, chilli flakes, garlic and chopped rosemary.

3 In a second bowl combine the Parmesan and the breadcrumbs. (If using only Parmesan, mix just half the Parmesan with the breadcrumbs.)

4 Preheat the oven to 200°C/400°F. Lightly oil a medium gratin dish.

5 Arrange a layer of steamed fennel slices in the base of the dish. Sprinkle over half the spicy oil and the pecorino. Cover with a second layer of fennel and sprinkle with the remaining spicy oil. Top with the Parmesan and breadcrumbs mix.

6 Cook the gratin in the top of the oven for 15–20 minutes. It should come out nicely browned on top and sizzling.

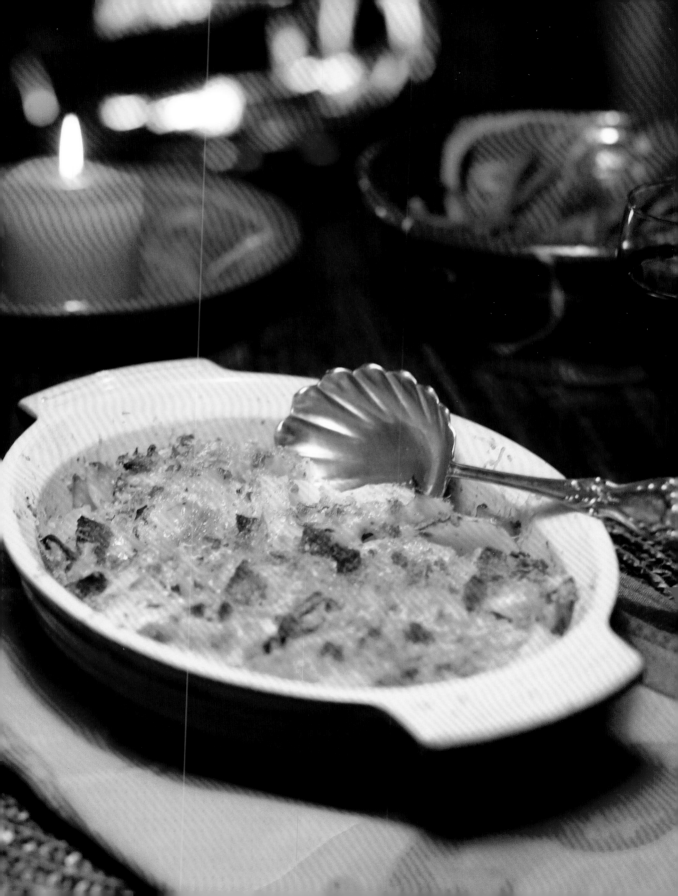

Autumn is the squash season. Butternut squashes dress modestly in light fawn, leaving their showier cousins – pumpkin, spaghetti squash, and so on – in yellow and red to hog the limelight around this time of year. Under the skin, though, they show their true colours. A wonderful autumn glow emerges, mustardy yellow – warming heart and body.

This recipe is adapted from one by Martha Rose Shulman in the New York Times. We usually finish the lot between us.

roasted butternut squash

SERVES 4

1kg/2lb 4oz butternut squash, peeled, deseeded and cut into small chunks

4 garlic cloves, finely chopped

1 tbsp wholegrain breadcrumbs

1 heaped tbsp chopped flat-leaf parsley

1 tbsp thyme leaves

3 tbsp olive oil

salt and freshly ground black pepper

1 Preheat the oven to 190°C/375°F.

2 Combine all the ingredients in a large bowl and mix them thoroughly together, seasoning well with salt and pepper.

3 Tip the mixture into a lightly oiled roasting tray and roast in the middle of the oven for about 50 minutes – the exact time depends on the size of the chunks – until the squash comes out nicely charred on top.

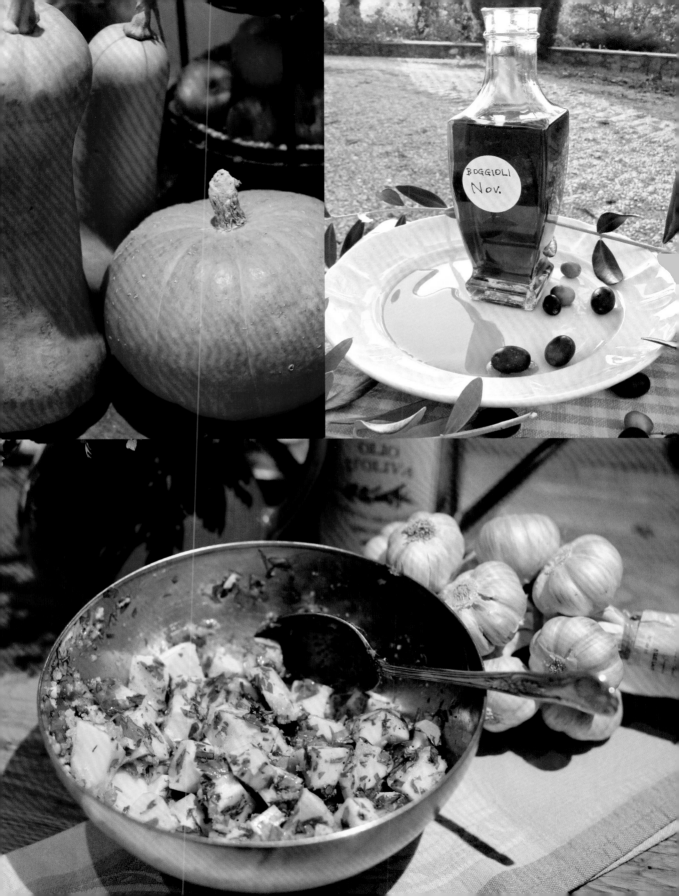

Our friends Helen and Keith live in the Chianti hills southeast of Florence (see p.108). They are olive farmers and are surrounded by a thousand olive trees. Helen is a natural cook. She rarely uses recipe books; rather, she builds a dish from the ingredients to hand – throwing in this and that with an instinctive sense of when it's right. I love watching her cook. She prepared this pasta on our visit last year – a reviving lunch after a morning working in the olive grove. It was creamy and delicious, and I found it hard not to take another spoonful. It seems to get better and better just sitting on the table. How did she manage to make it turn out that way? I asked her to cook it again for us this November – while I took notes.

helen's zucchini pasta

SERVES 4

3 tsp salt, plus more to taste, if necessary

3 tbsp olive oil

2 garlic cloves, crunched under a knife and roughly chopped

750g/1lb 10oz courgettes, sliced evenly

a pinch of cayenne powder

a handful of flat-leaf parsley, chopped

400g/14oz wholewheat penne, pasta spirals or shape of your choice

Parmesan cheese (optional), to serve

1 Set a large pan of water to boil over a high heat. Add 2 teaspoons of the salt.

2 Meanwhile, heat the oil in a large sauté pan over a low heat and add the garlic. Cook for 2–3 minutes, letting it take on some colour. Then add the courgette slices and a tablespoon of hot water, shaking the pan to coat the courgettes in the oil. Sprinkle over 1 teaspoon of the salt.

3 Leave the mixture to cook gently over a lowish heat, jiggling the pan from time to time, for about 20–25 minutes. Towards the end of the cooking time, add a little more salt if needed and add the cayenne and parsley.

4 Cook the pasta to just before al dente, then drain it, reserving a mugful of the cooking water. Add the drained pasta to the courgettes, then add a couple of spoonfuls of the reserved cooking water. Turn the pasta in the mixture, allowing the water to evaporate and the courgettes to take on a creaminess. (Helen keeps adding tablespoons of cooking water until the desired creaminess is achieved.)

5 Cover the pan until you're ready to serve, with a grating of Parmesan, if you wish (Helen leaves it as it is).

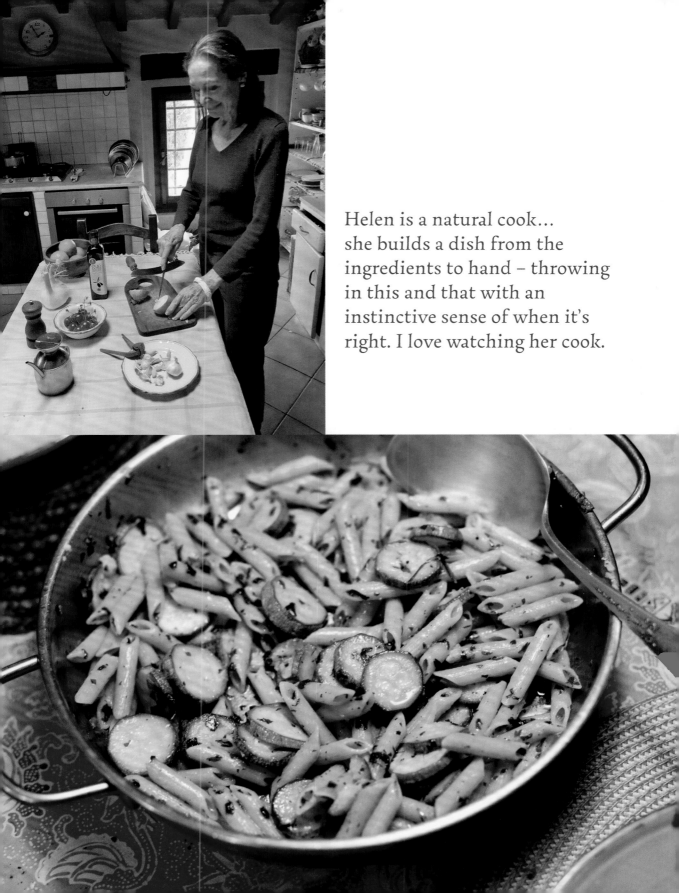

Helen is a natural cook…
she builds a dish from the
ingredients to hand – throwing
in this and that with an
instinctive sense of when it's
right. I love watching her cook.

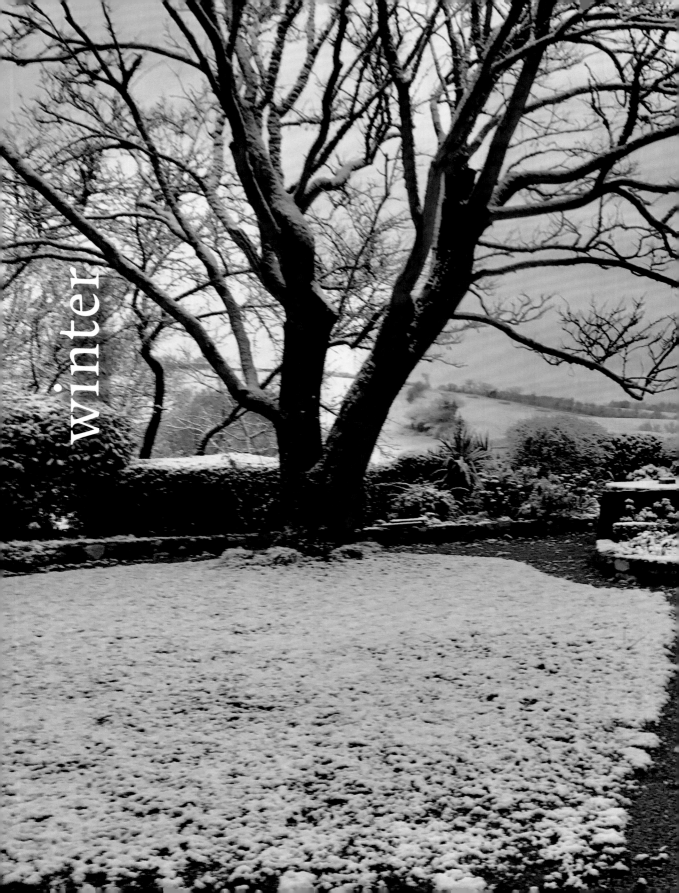

winter

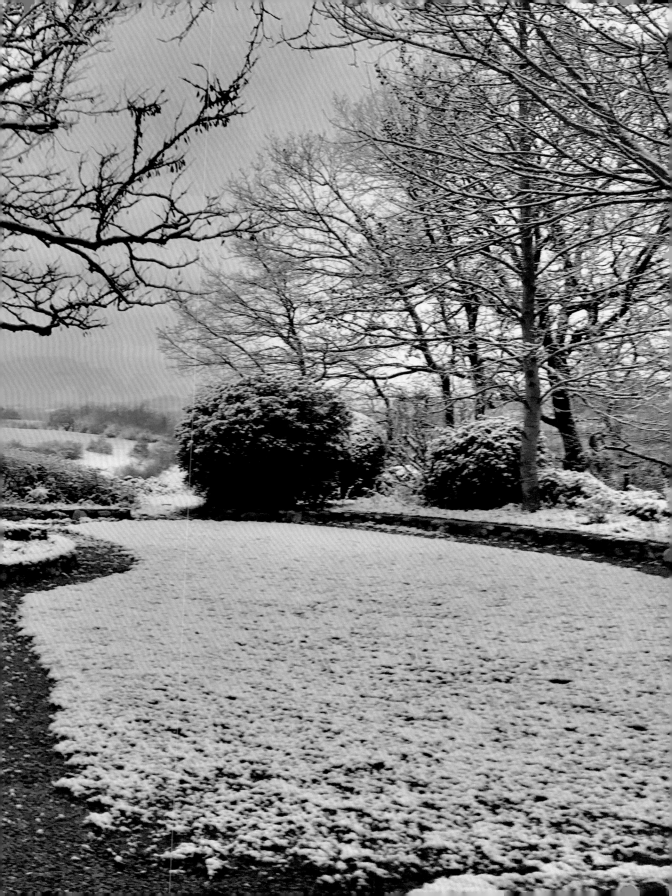

Now is the winter of our discontent / made glorious summer by this ... sun of February

I'm writing this on the last day of an extraordinary February. Winter has still three weeks to run and already we are seeing daffodils and irises showing their spring faces and the big willow on the back road to Lautrec in green cascade. Three weeks of blue sky and sun is causing some confusion in the natural world. We are enjoying our unseasonal lunches in the courtyard under the parasol and wearing sunglasses, but assuredly it will not last.

Winter still dominates on the market stalls and those lovely piles of white and green asparagus – our region of Occitania produces 25 per cent of France's yield each year – won't arrive for a couple of months. So winter remains on the table and in the kitchen and I'm not quite ready for a change.

Broccoli and fennel, white beans and lentils, red cabbage and cauliflower are enjoying the limelight and are not about to leave the stage. The versatile butternut squash is holding its ground and giving us some tasty suppers. Winter stuff and I like it – in winter!

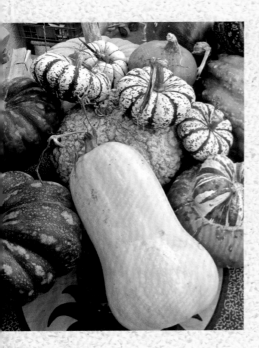

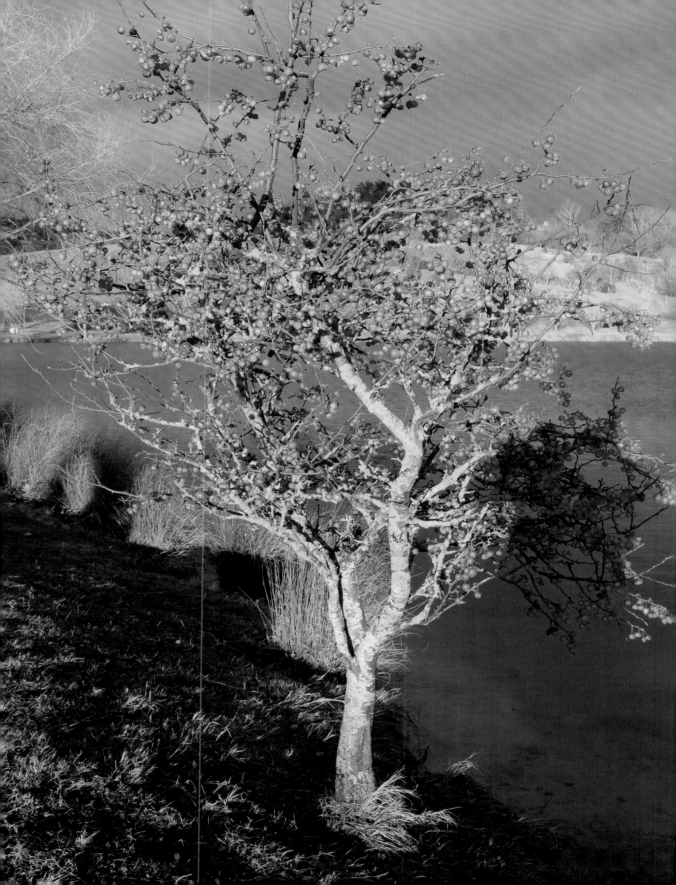

I made this soup the other night at Meredith's prompting. I was not feeling 100 per cent. She said this would serve me better than the windy bean and cabbage soup I was proposing (page 118 – a wondrously robust winter belter of a soup). She was right. I slept well and felt better in the morning.

It is simply a soup made with vegetables – no pulses, pasta or chickpeas. I like its simplicity and the taste (even better on the second day!).

vegetable soup

SERVES 4

2 tbsp olive oil

1 onion, chopped into small dice

1 leek, finely chopped

3 garlic cloves, crushed

3 carrots, 1 chopped into small dice,
2 into bite-sized dice

3 celery sticks, 1 chopped into small
dice, 2 into bite-sized dice

1 fennel bulb, chopped into
bite-sized dice

1 turnip, chopped into bite-sized dice

230g/8oz butternut squash, deseeded
and chopped into bite-sized dice

400g/14oz tin of plum tomatoes,
roughly chopped with juice

1 bay leaf, 2 sprigs parsley and
2 sprigs thyme, tied together

1.1 litres/4½ cups vegetable stock

salt and freshly ground black pepper

1 Heat the oil in a large saucepan over a lowish heat and add the onion, leek and garlic and the small-diced carrot and celery stick. Turn everything over in the oil and cook until tender. This is the taste engine of the soup that will slowly broadcast its deep tastiness through the rest of the cooking process.

2 Add all the bite-sized vegetables and the tomatoes and their juice and turn to combine. Then, add the tied herbs and the stock and season lightly with salt and pepper. Bring everything up to the boil, cover with a lid and reduce the heat to low. Simmer for 30 minutes, until the bite-sized vegetables are tender. Remove the tied herbs before serving.

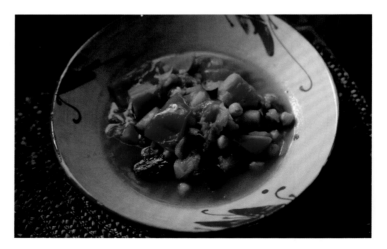

A good soup to cook, as I am doing, on New Year's Day morning after a prolonged night of celebration. It's also a good soup to try out if you have convinced yourself you can't cook – just stick it all in a pot and let it simmer.

I'm reminded by a friend that it's an Italian custom to cook lentils on this day. Their shape suggests coins and thus prosperity and good luck. We are going to Rome for my birthday later this week. A happy start to the year.

super simple lentil soup

SERVES 4

300g/10oz puy or green lentils

3 carrots, chopped

1 fennel bulb, damaged outer layers removed, chopped

3 tomatoes, fresh or tinned, chopped

3 shallots, chopped

3 garlic cloves, pulped with a pinch of salt

750ml/3 cups vegetable stock

1 bay leaf and a sprig of thyme, tied together with string

3 tbsp chopped flat-leaf parsley

8 pitted green olives

8 pitted black olives

1 tbsp tomato concentrate, from a tube or small tin

1 tsp salt

2 tbsp olive oil

zest of 1 lemon

freshly ground black pepper

1 Put all the ingredients except the oil and lemon zest in a large saucepan and season with a good few grindings of black pepper. Bring to the boil, then reduce the heat to a low simmer.

2 Cook covered for 30 minutes, or until the vegetables are tender. Stir in the oil and lemon zest and serve hot. *Buon appetito! e Buon anno!*

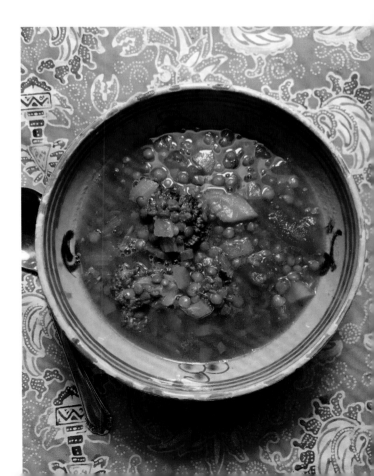

A winter soup that is satisfying to make on a cold, rainy afternoon. There is not a lot of work involved; most of the time the soup chugs away on its own, on top of the stove – I'm writing this while it chugs. The recipe is adapted from one by the inimitable Marcella Hazan.

red cabbage soup – 'the chugger'

SERVES 4

8 tbsp olive oil

½ onion, chopped

4 garlic cloves, 2 chopped and 2 pulped

1 tsp smoked paprika

1 tsp thyme leaves or a pinch of dried thyme

3 tomatoes, fresh or tinned (tinned are best this time of the year), chopped with their juice

450g/1lb red cabbage, quartered, cored and roughly sliced

1 celery stick, chopped

1½ tsp salt

590ml/2½ cups vegetable stock

about 500g/18oz jar or tin of white beans, drained

1 tsp very finely chopped rosemary

1 Gently heat half the oil in a large saucepan. Add the onion, chopped garlic, smoked paprika and thyme and sauté for about 10 minutes, until they start to take on some colour. Add the tomatoes, cabbage and celery, and mix thoroughly. Cook for about 30 minutes, until the cabbage has softened completely.

2 Stir in the salt and stock, cover the pan with a lid and cook on a very low heat for 2 hours (or longer, if you like!). This is the chugging stage (you'll hear it – chug-chug).

3 Separate half the beans into a bowl and add a little of the liquid from the soup. Using a stick blender, purée the beans in the bowl then add them to the pan with the vegetable mixture. Cook for 10 minutes, covered, to heat through, then stir in the remaining beans. Cover the pan again and let the soup chug-chug for 10–15 minutes longer.

4 Now the authentic Italian bit! Gently heat the remaining 4 tablespoons of oil in a small frying pan. Add the pulped garlic and cook for 2 minutes until lightly coloured. Remove the pan from the heat and add the chopped rosemary.

5 Pour this flavoured oil through a metal sieve into the soup. On a low heat, cook for a further 10 minutes, lid on, for the flavours to mingle before serving.

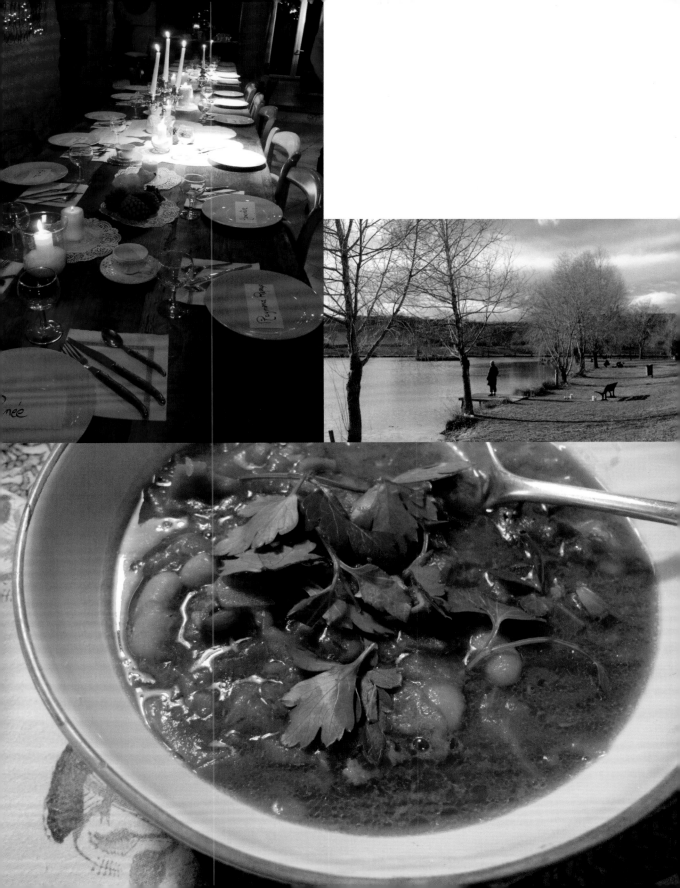

Cheating here on the seasonal theme, but this light and bright salad did cheer up a gloomy end-of-winter day and remind us that there are blue skies on the horizon. You don't need much of this little wonder, which is chock full of fibre. The white variety of quinoa will show off the red and yellow of the peppers better than the red or black.

quinoa salad with red and yellow peppers

SERVES 2 OR 3

100g/3½oz white quinoa, rinsed

200ml/generous ¾ cup vegetable stock

2 tbsp olive oil

1 red pepper, peeled, deseeded and chopped into large dice

1 yellow pepper, peeled, deseeded and chopped into large dice

1 garlic clove, pulped with a pinch of salt

½ tsp ground coriander

1 tbsp chopped coriander or flat-leaf parsley

1 small red or sweet onion, sliced

6 cherry tomatoes, quartered and deseeded

For the lemon vinaigrette

1 tbsp lemon juice

3 tbsp olive oil

salt and freshly ground black pepper

1 Put the quinoa in a small saucepan with the stock, and place over a low to medium heat. Bring to the simmer, then cover and cook for about 15 minutes, until the liquid has evaporated and the quinoa is tender.

2 Meanwhile, heat the olive oil in a large sauté pan, add the peppers, garlic and ground coriander and gently soften them for about 15 minutes without burning. Cover for part of the time to encourage the process.

3 To make the vinaigrette, put the lemon juice and olive oil in a screwtop jar. Season with salt and pepper, secure the lid and shake well to combine.

4 When the quinoa is ready, add the pepper and garlic mixture along with the fresh herbs and turn to combine. Add 1 tablespoon of the vinaigrette. Use the remaining 2 tablespoons of vinaigrette to dress the tomatoes and sliced onions. Top the quinoa with this little salad.

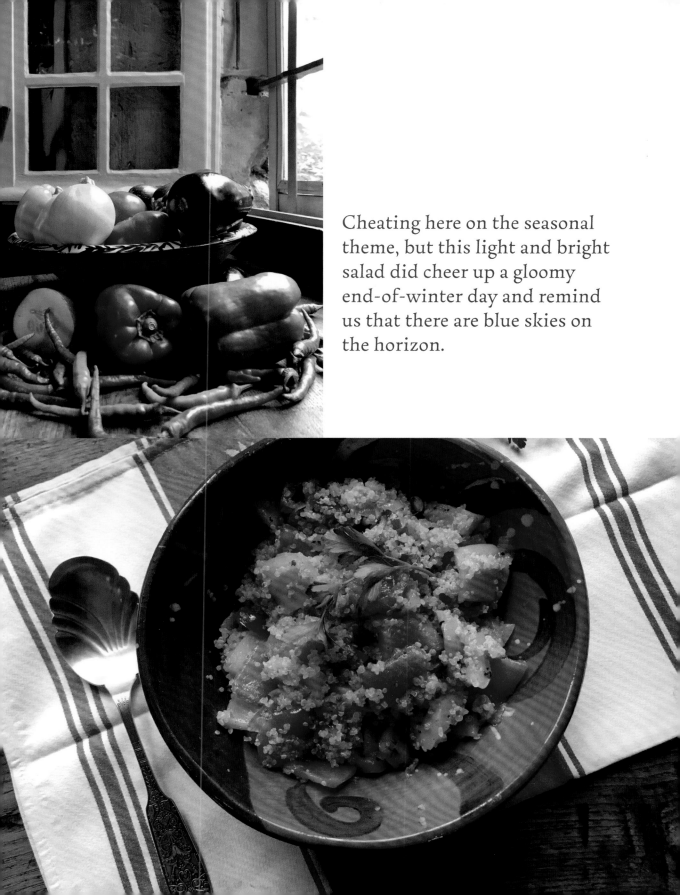

Cheating here on the seasonal theme, but this light and bright salad did cheer up a gloomy end-of-winter day and remind us that there are blue skies on the horizon.

Thin slices of apple, fennel and radish and nobbly nuts make this a useful early winter salad. For presentation, a sprinkling of chopped parsley helps.

fennel, apple, radish, walnut and pecorino salad

SERVES 2 OR 3

1 tbsp lemon juice

3 tbsp olive oil

1 apple, peeled and sliced as thin as can be

1 fennel bulb, outer leaves removed, halved and sliced as thin as can be

a handful of radishes, sliced as thin as you can without losing the skin on your finger or thumb

pecorino Romano, sliced as thin as you can (the amount is your choice, but remember that pecorino is salty)

a handful of walnut halves

chopped flat-leaf parsley

salt and freshly ground black pepper

1 Put the lemon juice and olive oil in a screwtop jar. Season with salt and pepper, secure the lid and shake to combine to a dressing.

2 Arrange the slices of apple and fennel on a salad dish and sprinkle over the slices of radish and pecorino. Set aside.

3 Place the walnut halves in a dry frying pan on a lowish heat and toast until they start to colour. Tip the toasted walnuts into the salad, then add some chopped parsley.

4 Pour over the dressing and turn everything carefully to combine.

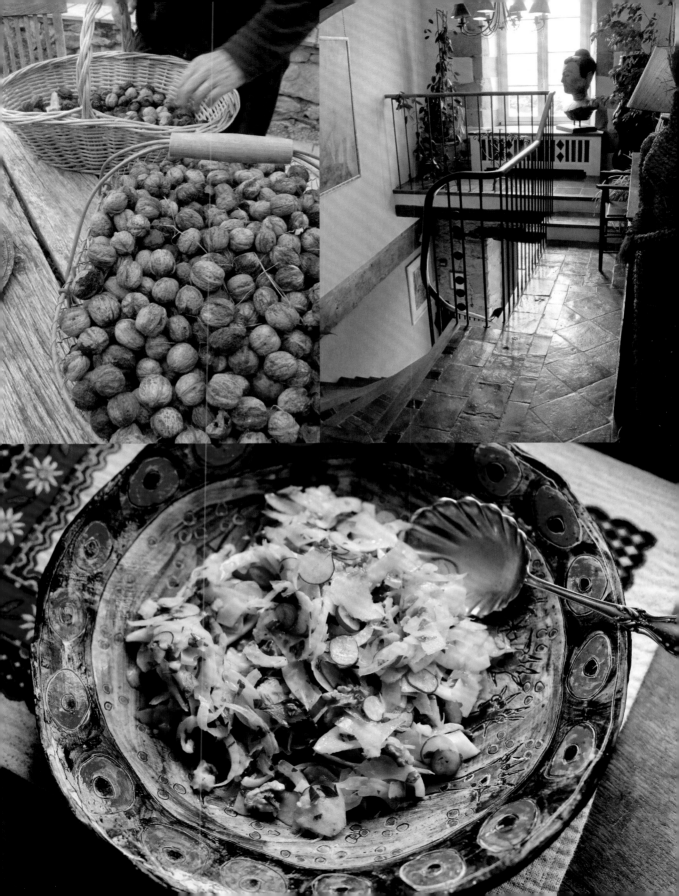

Farro is an ancient grain now grown most commonly in the mountainous area of northeast Tuscany. It has a pleasingly chewy texture and serves well as a base for salads in summer and winter as well as risotto-like recipes. Barley would be a substitute but it's worth 'foraging' for farro. What you include is an open choice: leftover cooked winter vegetables, revived by grilling or roasting, can be handy. Roasted hazelnuts and shavings of pecorino expand the flavours. The orange of the butternut squash and green of the Swiss chard brighten up the table.

farro salad with roasted winter veg

SERVES 2 OR 3

450ml/1¾ cups vegetable stock

250g/9oz farro

340g/12oz butternut squash, peeled, deseeded and cut into small dice

2 tbsp olive oil

1 large shallot, chopped

120g/4oz Swiss chard, sliced in small strips

50g/2oz pecorino shavings

50g/2oz hazelnuts, roasted (see p.120)

salt and freshly ground black pepper

For the dressing

1 tbsp balsamic vinegar

3 tbsp olive oil

1 Preheat the oven to 200°C/400°F.

2 Pour the stock into a large saucepan and add the farro. Bring to the boil, turn down the heat to low and cook for 30 minutes until tender but retaining a nice chewiness. Drain and set aside.

3 Toss the butternut squash in half the olive oil then spread it over a shallow baking tray. Cook in the oven for 25 minutes, until tender and beginning to brown.

4 Meanwhile, heat the remaining oil in a lidded pan and add the shallot. Fry over a lowish heat until softened. Add the Swiss chard, turn it over in the mix, then cover and cook for 5–7 minutes, until tender. It should melt in the mouth.

5 Add the cooked farro, butternut squash and the cheese and mix together.

6 Combine the ingredients for the dressing and pour it over the salad while it is still warm. Scatter the roasted hazelnuts over the top before serving, warm or at room temerature. Season with salt and pepper and turn it all over carefully.

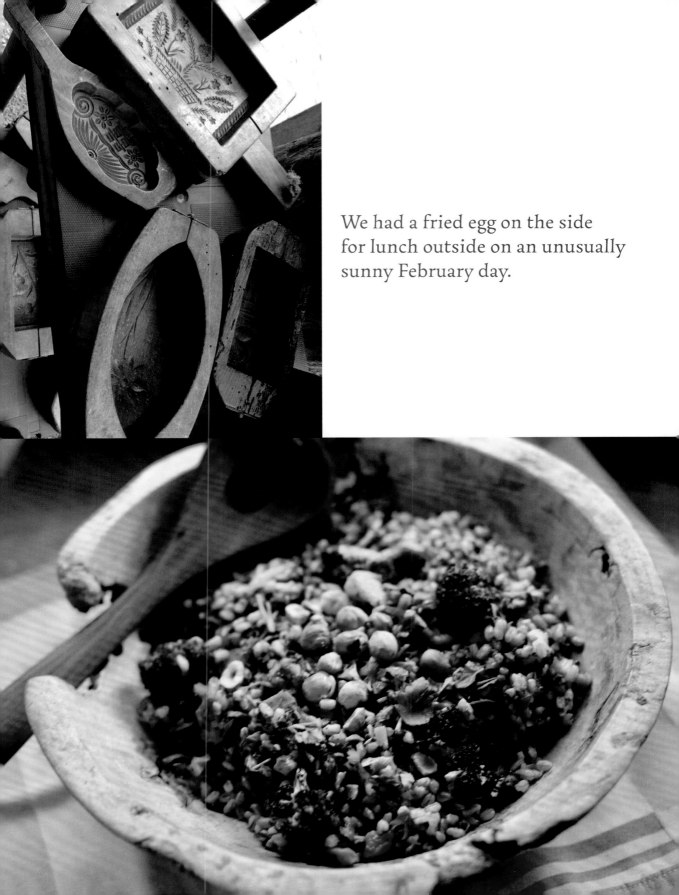

We had a fried egg on the side
for lunch outside on an unusually
sunny February day.

We had these for lunch on a sunny February day with grilled sucrines (little gem lettuces – see p.44) and the mushroom stalks sautéed on the side. Quite cheered us up. You have to have the spinach pesto to hand, but it serves as a useful everyday sauce and keeps its brilliant green colour better than its summer basil-based cousin.

mushrooms stuffed with baby spinach pesto

SERVES 4

250g/9oz ricotta

2 tbsp Baby Spinach Pesto (see p.207)

5 tbsp olive oil

8 large mushrooms, stalks removed and reserved

4 tbsp grated Parmesan if needed

2 tbsp chopped flat-leaf parsley

1 Preheat the oven to 200°C/400°F.

2 In a bowl, lightly mix together the ricotta and the pesto with a fork.

3 Brush an ovenproof dish – big enough to take all the mushrooms in one layer – with 1 tablespoon of the oil.

4 Arrange the mushroom cups in the dish. Spoon equal amounts of the ricotta and pesto mixture into each mushroom, filling generously (I find a teaspoon is best for this). Sprinkle over the Parmesan and drizzle over the remaining oil.

5 Bake for about 20 minutes, until the mushrooms have softened nicely and the top has browned a little. Sprinkle over the parsley and serve hot or at room temperature.

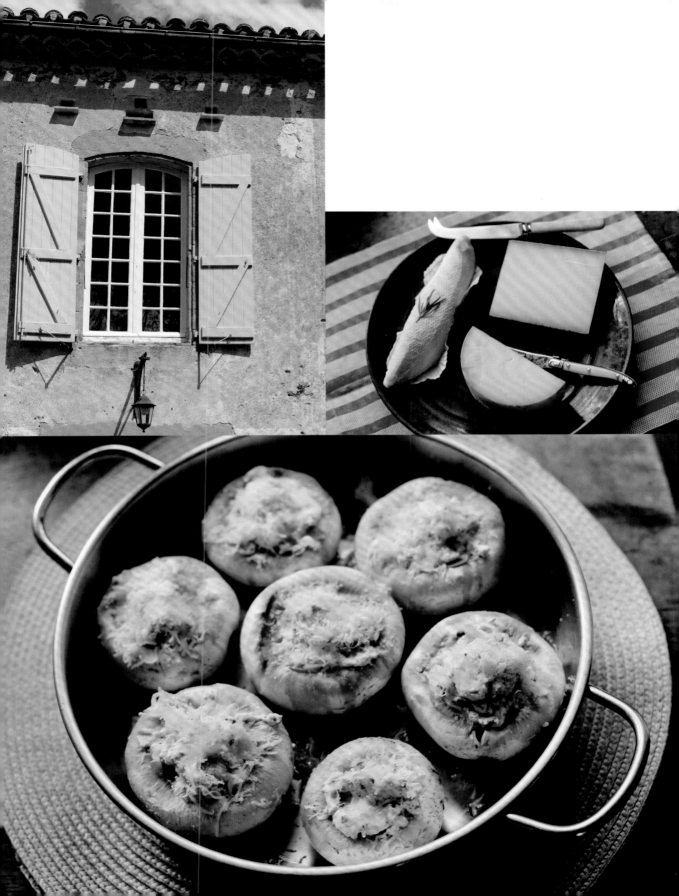

This frittata is the simplest I know and a joy to behold. Strong yellows and greens mix with the red of the onion. It is a cheery sight on a wet and windy winter's day.

broccoli frittata

SERVES 4

2 tbsp olive oil

1 red onion, sliced

450g/1lb broccoli, broken into bite-sized florets

5 eggs, beaten

50g/2oz Parmesan, grated

salt and freshly ground black pepper

1 Heat a tablespoon of the olive oil in a small frying pan over a medium heat. Add the onion slices and sauté for about 10 minutes, until softened and starting to brown. Park them in a mixing bowl.

2 Steam the broccoli florets until tender – test them with the tip of a knife. Add them to the onion in the bowl, turn to mix and leave to cool.

3 When the broccoli pieces have cooled, mix in the beaten eggs and the Parmesan and season with salt and pepper.

4 Heat the remaining olive oil in a frying pan with a heatproof handle. When hot, add the broccoli and egg mixture, spreading it evenly over the base of the pan. Reduce the heat to its lowest setting and leave the frittata to cook for about 25 minutes, until just a small pool of egg remains uncooked in the centre.

5 Heat the grill to hot.

6 Place the frying pan under the hot grill for 2–3 minutes, taking care not to burn the top of the frittata or dry it out.

7 Remove from the grill and ease a heatproof spatula around the circumference of the pan. Gently push the spatula under the frittata to persuade it away from the base of the pan, then ease it out onto a serving plate.

8 Slice the frittata into four or eight equal pieces before serving.

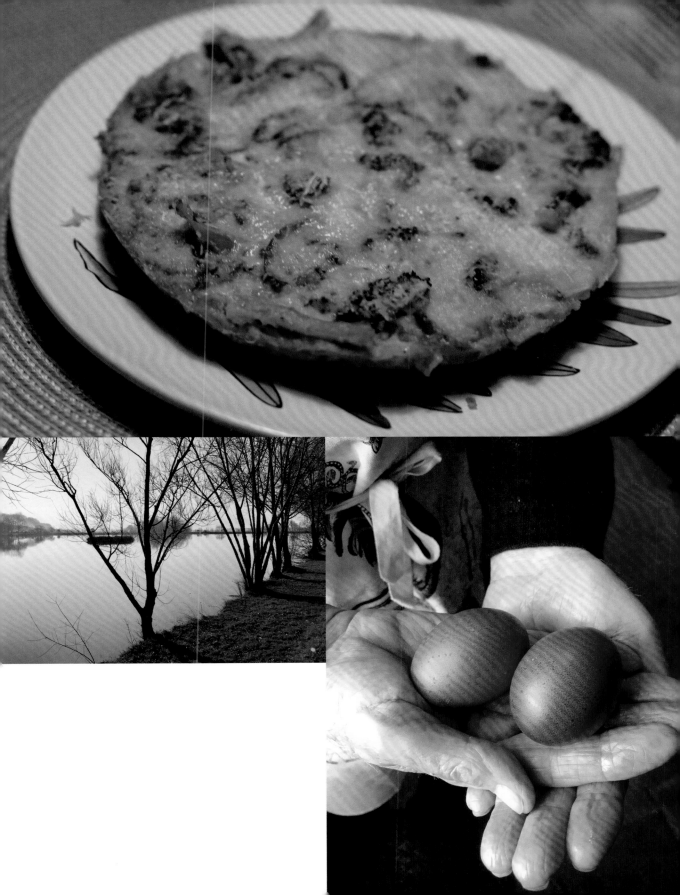

I like both the convenience and look of gratins. They often involve pre-cooked ingredients, so the final stage is a simple matter of heating through, which means you can do an assembly job beforehand. Then, you just heat the oven and hey presto! It's not the most photogenic dish, but scores highly on taste. The juicy black olives lend depth and an exotic twist.

cauliflower gratin with black olives

SERVES 2

1 cauliflower, broken into bite-sized florets

4 tbsp olive oil

1 onion, chopped

2 garlic cloves, pulped with a pinch of salt

2 tbsp finely chopped flat-leaf parsley

12 or so pitted juicy black olives, halved

4 tbsp grated Parmesan, or 2 tbsp each of Parmesan and pecorino Romano

2 tbsp wholegrain breadcrumbs

salt and freshly ground black pepper

1 Preheat the oven to 190°C/375°F.

2 Steam the cauliflower florets to your liking – I like them a bit firm – and set aside.

3 Heat 3 tablespoons of the oil in a large frying pan over a medium heat. Add the onion and sauté for about 5 minutes, until soft and browned a little.

4 Add the garlic and parsley and cook for another 2–3 minutes. Remove from the heat and mix in the olives. Add the cauliflower to the pan and turn it over in the mix, seasoning as you go with salt and pepper (don't over-salt if you're using pecorino, as it's already quite salty). Sprinkle over half the cheese and stir to mix. Taste for seasoning, adding more if necessary.

5 Place the mixture in a shallow gratin dish.

6 Mix the remaining cheese with the breadcrumbs and sprinkle over the mixture, then sprinkle over the remaining tablespoon of olive oil. Cook in the middle of the oven for about 20 minutes, until it is sizzling quietly and nicely browned on top. We ate it with a side of sautéed Brussels sprouts.

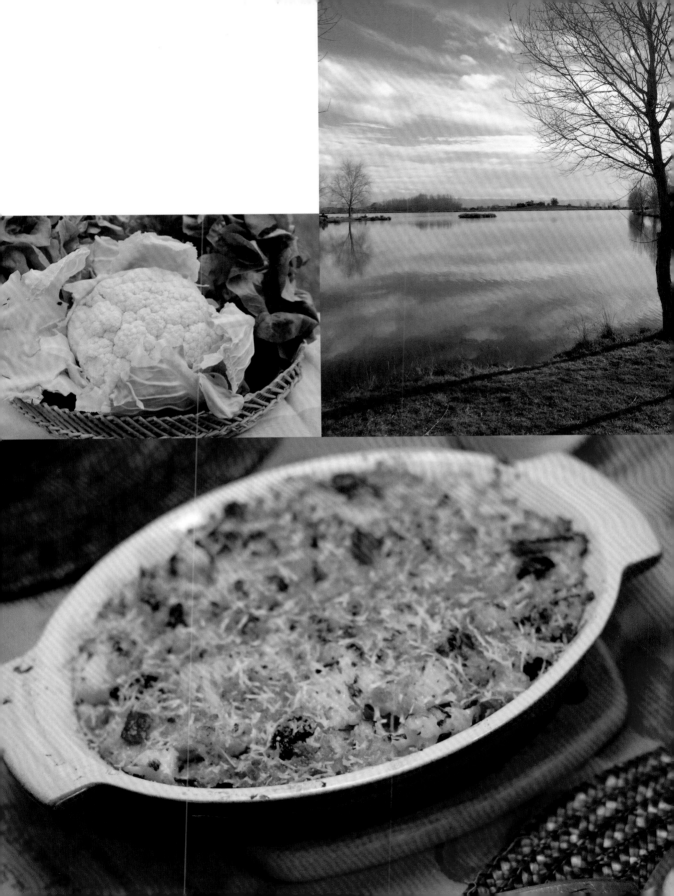

This is an evergreen standby for supper. Testing new stuffings is fine except testing requires tasting, and tasting can mean you've eaten dinner before teatime.

I have never been a fan of rice or grain fillings, so meaty mushrooms and fennel take the stage, mixed with garlic, parsley, black olives and onion or shallot. You might substitute walnuts for the black olives (Meredith says it's not easy to find good olives, so walnuts – dry-roasted – might be a more reliable choice) and some cooked broccoli for the fennel. I find peppers with four bumps at the base the easiest to halve.

winter stuffed peppers

SERVES 2

1 large fennel bulb, outer layers removed, quartered and chopped

4 tbsp olive oil, plus extra for brushing

1 medium onion, chopped

170g/6oz button mushrooms, quartered

1 garlic clove, chopped

a handful of flat-leaf parsley, chopped

10 meaty, pitted black olives, chopped

4 tbsp grated pecorino or Parmesan

2 red or yellow peppers, halved top to bottom, deseeded and white membrane removed

salt and freshly ground black pepper

1 Steam the fennel until tender, and set aside.

2 Heat 1 tablespoon of the oil in a frying pan and gently fry the onion for about 5 minutes, until it starts to colour. Remove from the pan and place in a bowl.

3 Fry the mushrooms in a second tablespoon of oil over a medium heat for about 5 minutes, until they start to colour.

4 Add the garlic and parsley and fry for a few seconds, stirring and taking care not to burn the garlic.

5 Add the mushrooms, garlic and parsley to the onion. Mix in the black olives and the fennel.

6 Sprinkle over 3 tablespoons of the cheese and mix it in, then season to taste. *Voila!* You have your stuffing. Set aside.

7 Now, for the peppers. Preheat the oven to 200°C/400°F. Line an oven tray with foil and brush lightly with oil.

8 Place the empty pepper halves on the oiled foil and sprinkle with a third tablespoon of oil. Place in the top half of the oven and roast for 20 minutes.

9 Remove from the oven and fill each pepper with a good spoonful of the stuffing mixture.

10 Top the peppers with the remaining cheese and sprinkle with the remaining tablespoon of olive oil.

11 Return them to the top half of the oven for another 20 minutes. They will be a bit charred and sizzling.

12 If the peppers still seem on the tough side when pierced with the point of a knife, cook them a little longer. It's a judgement call; you don't want to incinerate the stuffing.

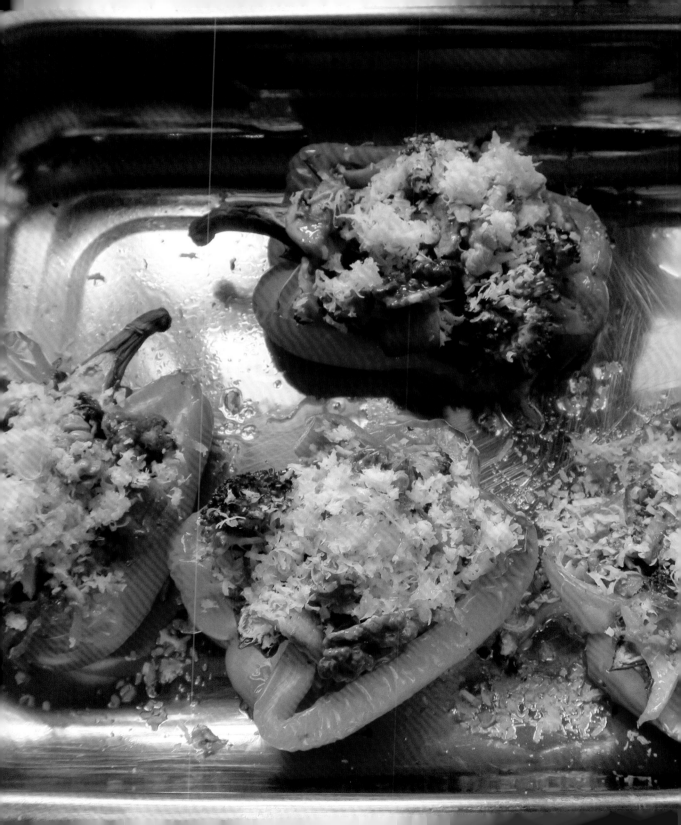

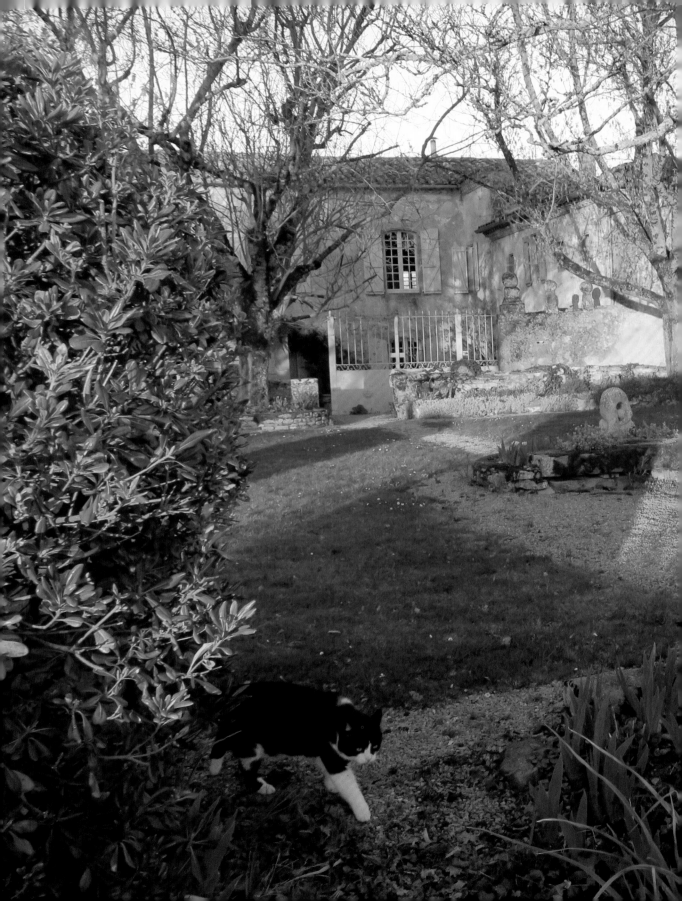

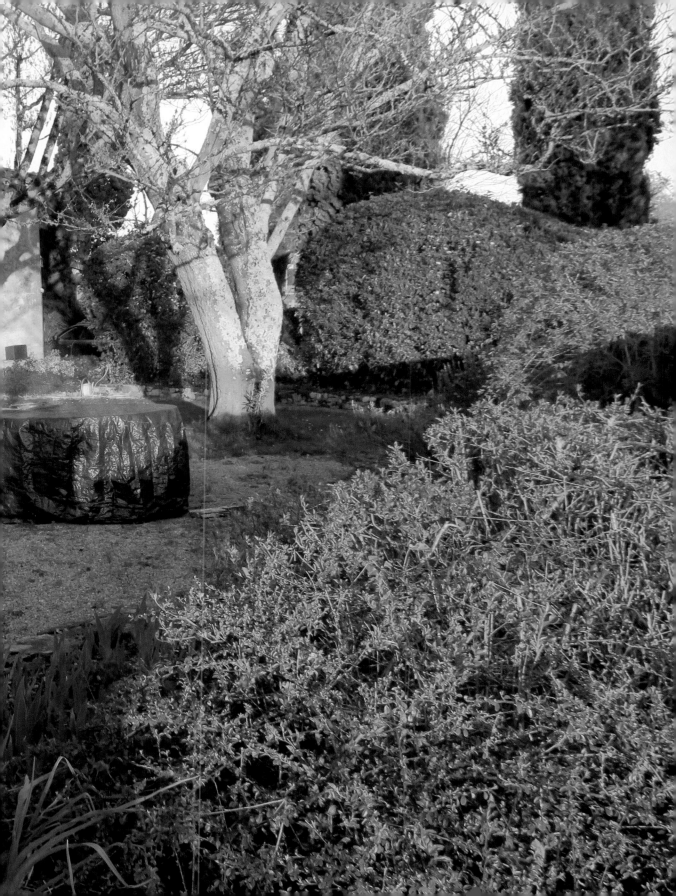

I make this using artichoke hearts from a jar, bought on a trip to Tuscany. It reminds me of countless lunches eaten at Trattoria Sostanza in Florence, a little eaterie discovered by chance on a trip in 1977 and unchanged 40 years later. I always order artichoke omelette, served flat, and a plate of white beans with olive oil.

artichoke omelette

MAKES 2 OMELETTES

2 tbsp chickpea flour, seasoned with salt and pepper

240g/9oz tin or jar of cooked artichoke hearts, drained, sliced vertically and patted dry with kitchen paper

2 tbsp olive oil

4 eggs

2 tbsp grated Parmesan

salt and freshly ground black pepper

1 Place the seasoned chickpea flour on a plate. Tip the sliced artichokes into the flour and turn over to lightly coat them.

2 Heat 1 tablespoon of the oil in an omelette pan over a lowish heat. Add the artichoke slices and fry gently until nicely browned on both sides. Remove from the pan and set aside.

3 Break two of the eggs into a bowl. Lightly beat them, then season with salt and pepper.

4 Turn up the heat under the pan and add the remaining oil. When hot, add the beaten egg, pushing back the liquid from the rim of the pan and letting it run into the spaces. Add half the artichokes, sprinkle over half the Parmesan and fold over the omelette. Slip the omelette out of the pan and onto a plate. Keep warm while you add a little more oil to the pan and repeat the process for the second omelette.

Adapted from a recipe by Ali Slagle in the New York Times, this is a delicious and useful gratin.

tomato-y white bean gratin

SERVES 4

1 tbsp olive oil, plus extra for drizzling

3 garlic cloves, crushed with a pinch of salt

1 tsp very finely chopped rosemary

3 tbsp tomato concentrate out of a tube or small tin

3 tbsp warm water

400g/14oz jar or tin of white beans, drained

30g/1oz Parmesan, grated

30g/1oz wholegrain breadcrumbs

salt and freshly ground black pepper

1 Preheat the oven to 200°C/400°F.

2 In a medium pan, heat the olive oil and sauté the garlic and rosemary over a low heat until the garlic starts to colour. Add the tomato concentrate and heat through gently. Stir in the warm water and fold in the beans, then season with salt and pepper, mixing well as you do so.

3 Transfer the mixture to an ovenproof dish and set aside.

4 In a small bowl, mix together the cheese and breadcrumbs, then sprinkle this over the bean mixture in the dish. Drizzle a little olive oil around the edge of the dish and back and forth across the dish.

5 Bake the gratin in the upper part of the oven for 10 minutes, or until it is nicely browned on top. Let it stand for 5 minutes before serving.

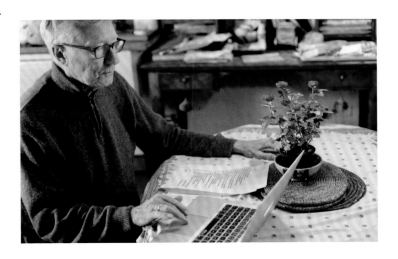

We had these the other night with roasted cabbage rounds (see p.197) and flageolet beans in a tomato sauce. The three made good company – rather than a crowd!

leeks in red wine

SERVES 4

4 leeks

3 tbsp olive oil

1 glass of red wine

2–3 tbsp vegetable stock, plus extra if necessary

salt and freshly ground black pepper

1 Cut off the root ends of the leeks and pull off any damaged outer layers. Peel back the tops a little to make sure the soil is cleaned away, then slice into stubby lengths.

2 Place the sliced leeks in a single layer in a pan (you'll need one with a lid). Add the oil and a pinch of salt and cook over a medium heat for about 7 minutes, until the leeks start to brown.

3 Turn them and add the wine and the stock (there'll be spluttering – be careful!). Cover the pan and cook on a medium heat for about 10–15 minutes, until the leeks are tender and the sauce is silkily viscous.

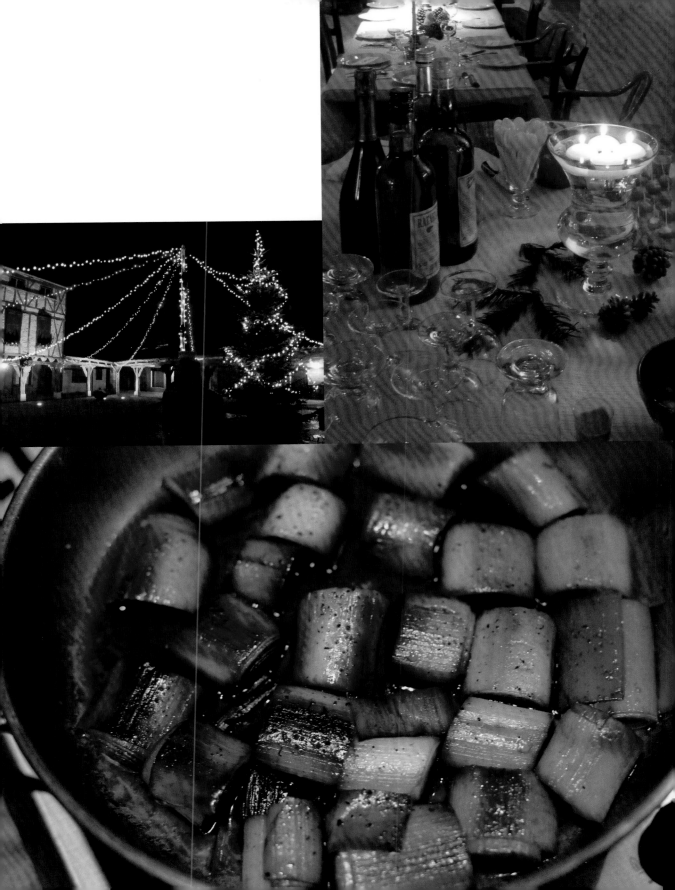

Fennel is the star turn; the supporting cast is for choice. Try mashing the turnip into the liquid. (When you buy coconut milk, it's wise to check the package – sweetened versions are an abomination.)

utterly delicious, mostly white winter vegetable gratin

SERVES 2 OR 3

2 tbsp olive oil

1 onion, chopped

2 garlic cloves, pulped with a pinch of salt

1 tsp smoked paprika

1 tsp finely chopped rosemary needles

2 fennel bulbs, outer parts removed, halved and sliced into bite-sized pieces

1 leek, damaged outer leaves removed, halved lengthways and sliced into bite-sized pieces

1 celery stick, sliced into bite-sized pieces

1 small turnip, peeled and cut into small bite-sized pieces

150ml/⅔ cup unsweetened coconut milk

150ml/⅔ cup vegetable stock

50g/2oz Parmesan or pecorino Romano, grated

salt and freshly ground pepper

1 Preheat the oven to 200°C/400°F.

2 Heat the oil in a shallow 22cm ovenproof pan over a medium heat. Add the onion and cook for 5 minutes, until it starts to soften. Add the garlic, smoked paprika and rosemary and cook for 2–3 more minutes, to soften further.

3 Add the rest of the bite-sized cast – the fennel, leek, celery and turnip – season with salt and pepper and stir to combine. Cook for a few minutes until the vegetables are softened, then add the coconut milk and stock.

4 Bring the mixture to the boil. Turn down the heat and sprinkle over the cheese.

5 Place the pan in the upper part of the oven for about 30 minutes, until it is nicely browned on top, checking after 20 minutes to make sure that the gratin isn't burning.

This winter stew is best when you stagger the way you add the ingredients – that way the potential mushers (the sweet potato or squash) stay in shape. It is straightforward but with a comforting kick.

simple spicy winter vegetable stew

SERVES 3 OR 4

1 tbsp olive oil, plus extra to serve

3 carrots, 1 diced very small and 2 cut into 2cm/¾in dice

1 onion, diced very small

2 celery sticks, 1 diced very small and 1 cut into 2cm/¾in dice

½ tsp ground cumin

½ tsp ground coriander

½ tsp hot smoked paprika

1 garlic clove, crushed in a mortar

½ tsp fennel seeds, pounded in a mortar

1 tsp tomato concentrate out of a tube or small tin

½ tsp harissa paste (optional)

250ml/1 cup vegetable stock

1 turnip, cut into 2cm/¾in dice

1 fennel bulb, outer leaves removed, halved and cut into 2cm/¾in dice

3 tbsp chickpeas from a tin

1 tsp salt

½ sweet potato, cut into 2cm/¾in dice (or 150g/5oz squash, if you prefer)

lemon juice, to serve

plain yoghurt or crème fraîche, to serve (optional)

1 Heat the olive oil in a casserole pan on a medium to low heat. Add the very small pieces of carrot, onion and celery and sauté for 6–7 minutes, until they begin to soften.

2 Add the spices, garlic, fennel seeds, tomato concentrate and, if using, the harissa. Let everything warm through and get to know each other for 3–4 minutes.

3 Fold in the remaining ingredients, except the sweet potato or squash, and bring up to the boil. Cover the pan and cook for about 10 minutes, then add the sweet potato or squash. Continue cooking, covered, for about 20 minutes, or until the vegetables are done to your taste. Serve with a squeeze of lemon juice and a swirl of olive oil or a dollop of yoghurt or crème fraîche.

A Greek take on the cauliflower, this dish is called kounoupidi kapama. The cinnamon here adds a delicate flavour, but be careful not to overdo it.

greek cauliflower in tomato and cinnamon sauce

SERVES 3 OR 4

4 tbsp olive oil

1 onion, finely diced

2 garlic cloves, pulped with a pinch of salt

1 cauliflower, broken into bite-sized florets

1 tsp ground cinnamon

250g/9oz tinned tomatoes, broken up a little

½ cinnamon stick

salt and freshly ground black pepper

1 Heat the oil in a saucepan over a medium heat. Add the onion and garlic and cook for 5 minutes, until softened.

2 Mix in the cauliflower pieces and cook until they soften and take on a little colour. Add the ground cinnamon, tomatoes and cinnamon stick along with 4 tablespoons of water and season with salt and pepper.

3 Turn everything over thoroughly, bring to the boil, then reduce the heat and cook gently for 15 minutes to meld the flavours and further tenderise the cauliflower.

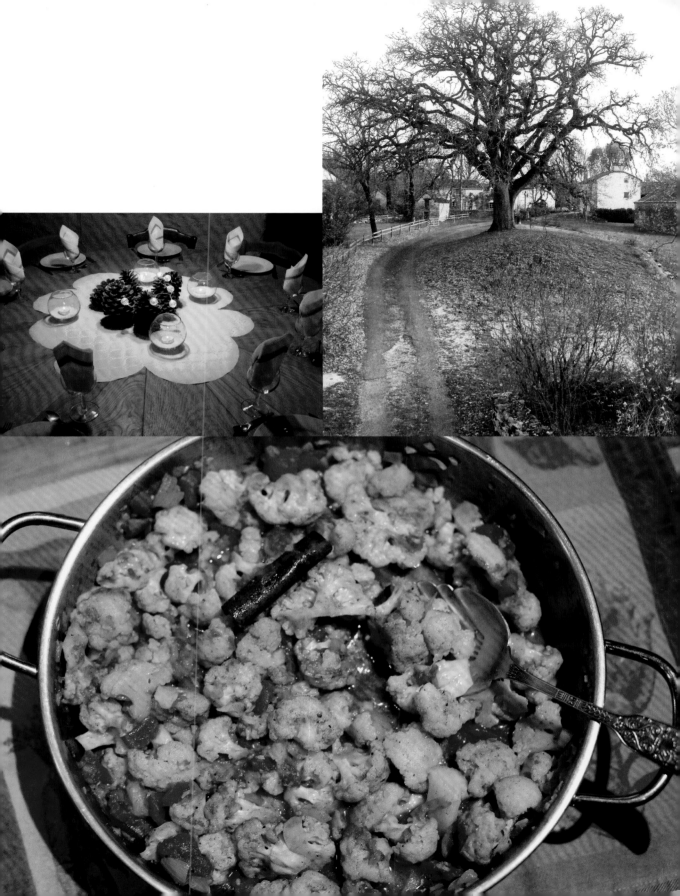

Although this recipe is often made using spinach, I prefer Swiss chard. It is more substantial and doesn't have the aftertaste of cooked spinach. A bunch each of green chard and red chard – if you can find the red and/or yellow sort – makes for a prettier dish.

swiss chard with eggs

SERVES 2

1 bunch each of green chard and red chard, leaves and stems separated

1 tbsp olive oil, plus extra for cooking the eggs

1 onion, chopped

1 garlic clove, chopped

½ tsp nutmeg

30g/1oz Parmesan, grated

4 eggs

1 Chop the chard stems into small dice and tear the leaves.

2 Cook the stems in boiling salted water for about 5 minutes, until tender, then remove them to a bowl, using a slotted spoon.

3 Add the leaves to the boiling water and cook for about 5 minutes, until tender. Remove as before.

4 Heat the oil in a large frying pan over a medium heat and add the onion and garlic. Fry for about 5 minutes, until softened. Add the chard leaves and stems and stir to mix. Add the nutmeg and cheese and mix in.

5 Cover the base of a small, lidded frying pan with olive oil. Place over a medium heat and add the chard mixture, spreading it out evenly. Carefully break the eggs on top of the mixture, cover the pan and cook over a medium heat until the eggs are cooked to your liking.

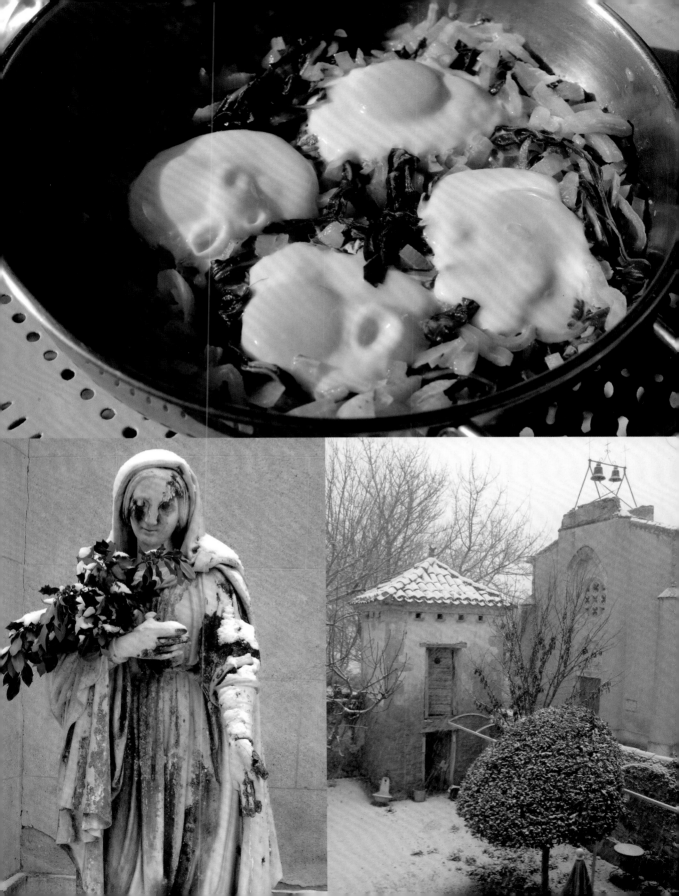

This is adapted from a recipe in Sirocco by Sabrina Ghayour, a lovely book of Persian cookery. The preserved lemons, if you can find them, and the apricots lend it authentic Middle Eastern flavours. The extra can of water is important as the butternut is a thirsty beast. The dish is best when there is plenty of sauce.

butternut squash tagine with chickpeas

SERVES 4

2 tbsp olive oil

2 onions, chopped

3 garlic cloves, chopped

1 tsp ground cinnamon

2 tsp ground cumin

1 tsp ground turmeric

500g/1lb 2oz butternut squash, peeled, deseeded and cut into 2cm/¾in pieces

400g/14oz tin of chickpeas, drained

peel of 2 preserved lemons

a handful of dried apricots

3 tsp harissa paste

400g/14oz tin of tomatoes, chopped

2 tsp salt

freshly ground black pepper

lemon wedges, to serve

1 Heat the olive oil in a large saucepan over medium to low heat. Add the onions and garlic and fry for 7–8 minutes, until they begin to colour. Stir in the cinnamon, cumin and turmeric.

2 Add the butternut squash, the chickpeas, the lemon peel and the apricots and turn everything over thoroughly, then mix in the harissa paste. Add the can of tomatoes and a further can of water, along with the salt. Season with a few turns of the peppermill.

3 Give it all a careful stir and leave to bubble gently for 30 minutes, stirring occasionally. (Add a little more water if necessary, being careful not to flood out the taste.) Serve with lemon wedges to squeeze over. Bulgur wheat goes well, too (see p.196).

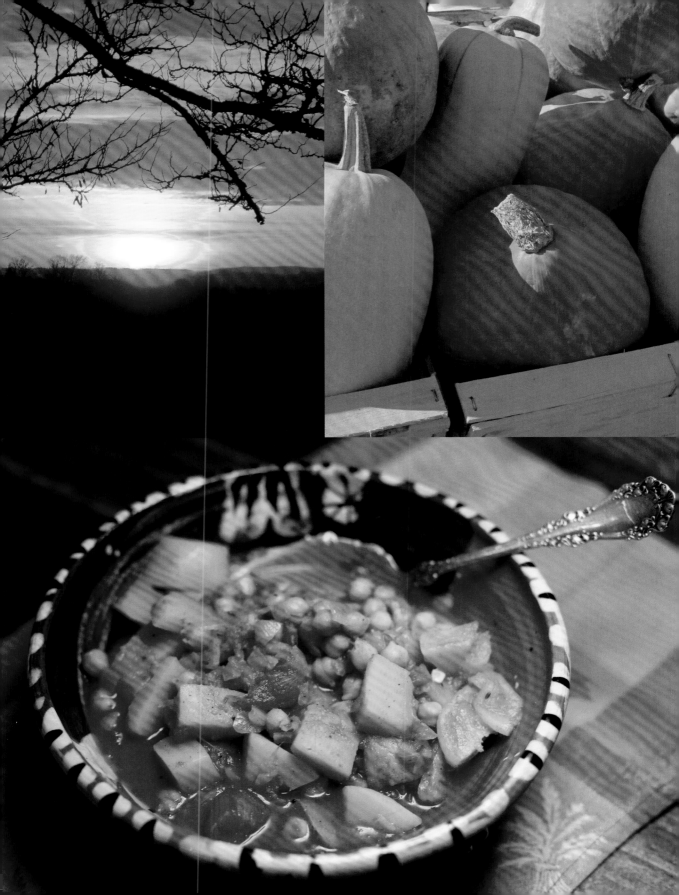

Bulgur has a slightly higher GI rating than rice and pasta but is still a useful alternative. Like them, it presents an empty canvas on which to paint using other ingredients.

bulgur with tomatoes, cinnamon and allspice

SERVES 2 OR 3

1 tbsp olive oil

1 small onion, finely chopped

300g/10oz tinned tomatoes, chopped

200g/7oz bulgur wheat

½ tsp ground cinnamon

½ tsp allspice

½ tsp salt

1 Heat the oil in a medium saucepan and gently soften the onion for about 7–8 minutes.

2 Add the tomatoes and stir them in thoroughly, then cover and cook for 5 minutes. Remove the lid and add the bulgur, spices and salt and stir in 300ml/1¼ cups of water. Bring to the boil, cover, and cook on a lowish heat for 10 minutes. Turn off the heat and let it stand, covered, for 15 minutes.

3 Fluff it up *et voilà* – you have a pinkish canvas.

Thick slices of green or white cabbage, infused with a simple marinade and roasted in the oven at a medium–high heat can serve as the main item on a lunch or dinner plate. They are a meaty eat – best to use a serrated steak knife. I favour the slightly looser-leafed green variety of cabbage for this dish.

The two-cheese version – with a topping of crumbled goat's cheese or feta on the Parmesan – got the DING from Meredith! A poached egg on top is a habit chez nous.

roasted cabbage rounds

SERVES 2

1 green or white cabbage, outer leaves removed

2 tbsp olive oil, plus extra for brushing

2 garlic cloves, pulped with a pinch of salt

2 tbsp lemon juice

freshly ground black pepper

4 tbsp grated Parmesan (or more, if desired)

1 Preheat the oven to 200°C/400°F.

2 Slice the cabbage into 2.5cm/1in slices – try to keep the same thickness as you slice, although this is a bit of a challenge.

3 Cover a shallow baking tray with foil and lightly brush it with oil. Arrange the cabbage slices on top.

4 Put the garlic, the 2 tablespoons of oil and the lemon juice into a screwtop jar. Season with pepper, then secure the lid and shake it all about. Use the mixture to generously brush the cabbage slices in the tray.

5 Cook in the middle of the oven for about 30 minutes, until nearly tender and starting to char. Take the tray out of the oven and use a fish slice to carefully turn over the slices.

6 Spread the Parmesan equally over the slices, then pop the tray back in the oven for 15 minutes, to brown the cheese nicely and further tenderise the slices.

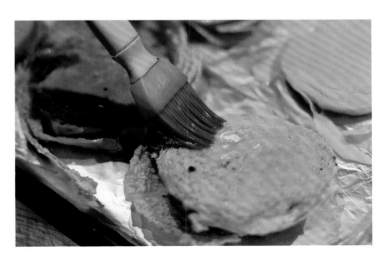

Serve this hot in a hand-warming bowl with a swirl of olive oil and it hits the spot.

swiss chard and white bean casserole

SERVES 4

700g/1½lb Swiss chard, leaves and
stalks separated

4 tbsp olive oil

1 onion, chopped

5 garlic cloves, chopped

2 tbsp chopped flat-leaf parsley

2 x 400g/14oz tins of white
beans, drained

250ml/1 cup vegetable stock

salt and freshly ground black pepper

1 Tear up the chard leaves into manageable pieces and slice the stalks finely.

2 Heat the oil in a deep pan over a medium-low heat. Add the onion and sauté for 7–8 minutes, until softened. Add the garlic and continue to cook for a couple of minutes, to soften.

3 Fold in the chard leaves, stalks and parsley and mix well with the garlicky oil, then add the beans and stock and season with salt and pepper. Bring the mixture up to a simmer and cook for about 20 minutes.

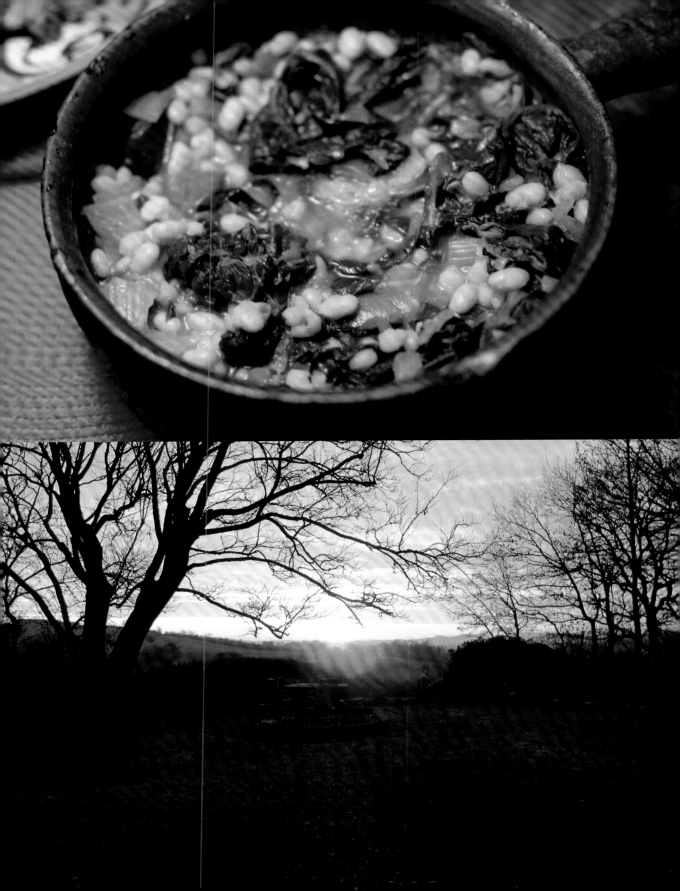

A steaming plate of freshly cooked broccoli with a small jug of olive oil to anoint it is a thing of beauty. This takes the cooked broccoli a couple of steps further without losing that particular broccoli taste.

sautéed broccoli with garlic

SERVES 4

2 tsp salt

500g/1lb 2oz broccoli, broken into bite-sized florets

3 tbsp olive oil

2 garlic cloves, pulped in a mortar with a pinch of salt

pinch of chilli flakes (optional)

pinch of chopped flat-leaf parsley (optional)

salt and freshly ground black pepper

1 Bring a saucepan of water to the boil and add the salt. Add the broccoli pieces and cook until just tender. You will need to test with the point of a knife after 2–3 minutes, while they are still a brilliant green. Drain and set aside.

2 Gently heat the oil in a large frying pan and add the garlic. Stir for 1 minute, then add the broccoli, and the chilli flakes and parsley, if using. Stir for a couple of minutes to heat through, then season to taste.

Cabbage is not to everyone's taste. The memory of school lunches – with cabbage cooked until it surrenders – is often a reason given for a lifetime's avoidance. But I love it and have just cooked and eaten half a small white cabbage that was lingering in the fridge.

simple white cabbage

SERVES 3 OR 4

1 small white cabbage,
outer leaves removed

olive oil and/or melted butter, or a
mixture (amount of your choice)

salt and freshly ground black pepper

1 Quarter the cabbage and cut out the tough stem. Cook the quarters in some well-salted boiling water for about 5 minutes, until just tender.

2 Remove the cabbage pieces with tongs and give them a good shake. Transfer them to a serving bowl and pour over the oil or melted butter (or mixture of both), then season with black pepper. Simplest thing in the world.

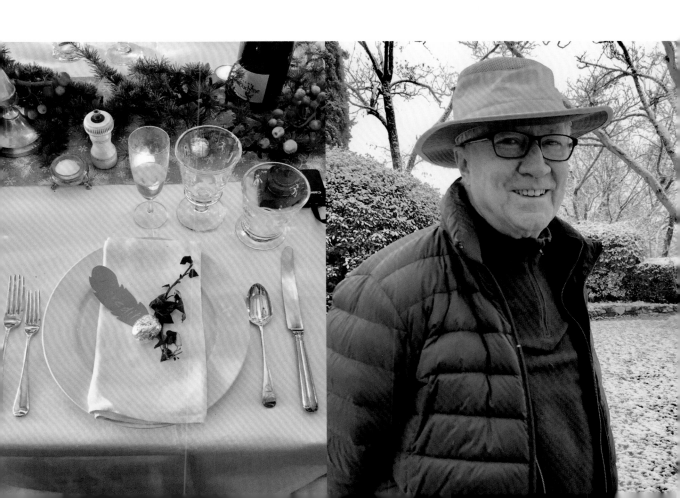

Broccoli pasta typically involves an anchovy sauce; this, of course, does not, but still manages to be scrummy.

broccoli pasta

SERVES 3 OR 4

450g/1lb broccoli, broken into
bite-sized florets

60g/2¼oz walnut pieces, broken up

5 tbsp olive oil

1 red onion, finely sliced

2 garlic cloves, finely sliced

2 small dried chillies, chopped

1 tsp fennel seeds, pounded
in a mortar

3 tbsp chopped flat-leaf parsley

12 juicy pitted black olives

300g/10oz wholewheat penne

50g/2oz pecorino Romano, grated,
plus extra to serve

1 Bring a saucepan of salted water to the boil and cook the broccoli for a few minutes until tender. Remove the broccoli with a slotted spoon and set aside, saving 100ml/scant ½ cup of the cooking water separately, to add to the sauce. Keep the rest of the water in the pan to cook the pasta later.

2 In a small frying pan, gently sauté the walnut pieces, dry, on a low heat, until they take on some colour, then set aside.

3 Heat 2 tablespoons of the olive oil in a shallow pan, large enough to hold the cooked pasta and broccoli later, over a medium heat. Add the onion and sauté until it starts to brown. Mix in the garlic, chillies and fennel seeds and cook for 1 minute, then add the parsley and the olives and cook for a further 2–3 minutes.

4 Add the cooked broccoli and the reserved cooking water and 3 tablespoons of olive oil. Break up the broccoli, stirring as it cooks, until it forms more of a sauce. Set aside.

5 Meanwhile, bring the broccoli water left in the saucepan to the boil. Add the pasta and cook according to the packet instructions or to your liking. Drain (reserving a little of the cooking water to add to the finished dish if you feel it needs easing a little), then stir it into the broccoli sauce in the shallow pan. Stir in the walnuts, then finally the cheese.

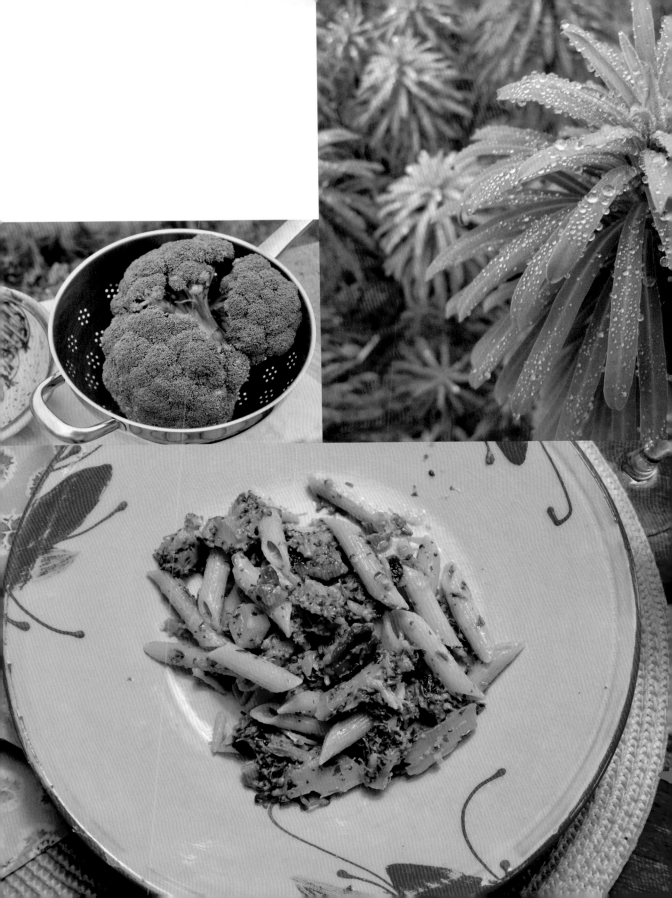

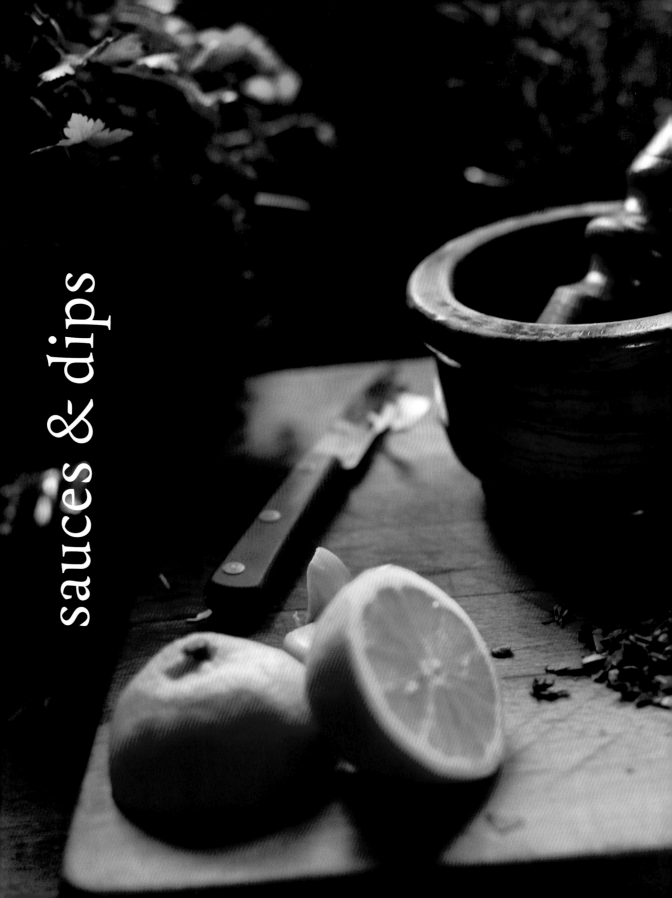

sauces & dips

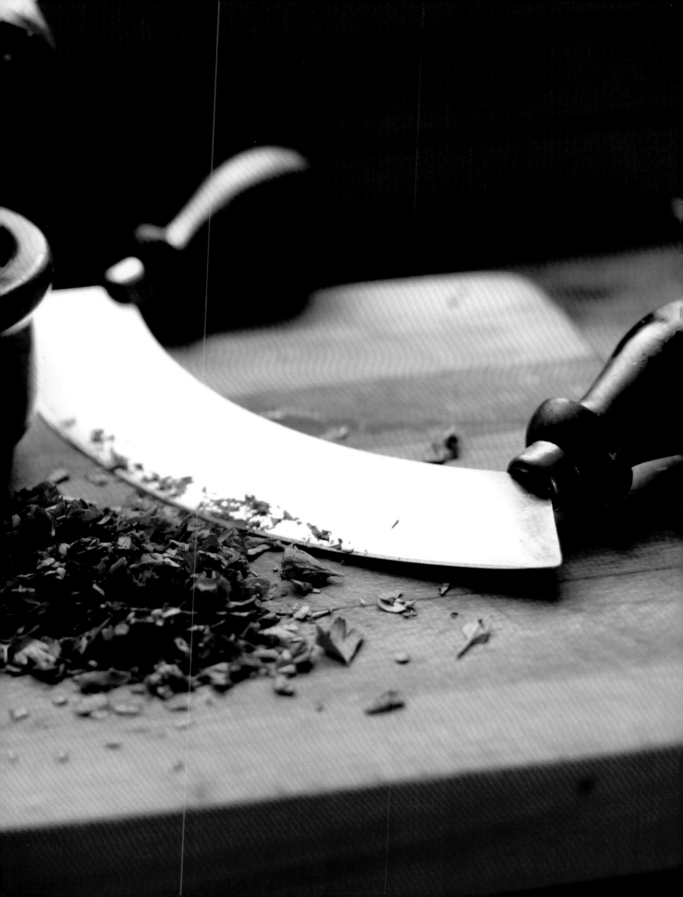

green olive and artichoke dip

SERVES 4

200g/7oz artichoke hearts from a jar, drained

5–6 tbsp olive oil

1 garlic clove, crushed with a pinch of salt

50g/2oz green olives, pitted

2 tbsp capers

3 tbsp chopped flat-leaf parsley

juice of 1 lime

salt and freshly ground black pepper

1 or 2 fennel bulbs, sliced, to serve

A nod to tapenade (see p.212), we first tasted this dip in Gail Zweigenthal's apartment overlooking Central Park when we were in New York recently. Gail was Editor-in-Chief of Gourmet magazine from 1991 to 1998, and this recipe featured.

Six simple ingredients plus seasoning make this a dip-in-a-flash. In fact, seven – Meredith thought a squeeze of lime or lemon juice would be good. The nod to tapenade comes with the capers. Caper in Provençal patois is tapinas.

1 Put all the ingredients except the seasoning and fennel slices in a food processor and whizz to a rough purée – leaving a little texture. Season to taste, and serve, as Gail did, on fennel slices or wholewheat toast with a dribble of olive oil.

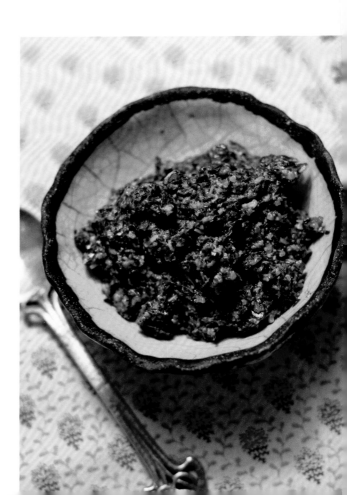

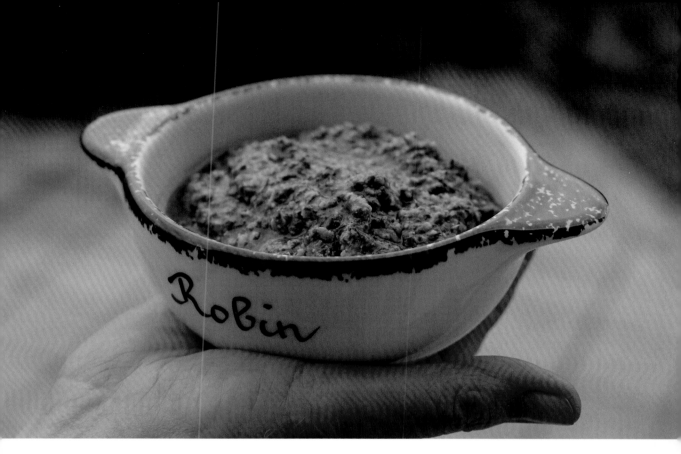

baby spinach pesto

SERVES 4

150g/5oz baby spinach,
stems removed

50g/2oz walnuts, lightly pan roasted

1 small garlic clove, crushed with a
pinch of salt

zest of 1 lemon, plus 2 tbsp juice

5 tbsp olive oil

50g/2oz Parmesan, grated,
or a mixture of pecorino Romano
and Parmesan

salt and freshly ground black pepper

A brilliantly green winter pesto – reassurance that spring is on its way. I have found that it keeps its colour handily in the fridge.

1 Put the spinach, walnuts, garlic, and lemon zest and juice in a food processor. Whizz to combine. With the motor running, add the oil, then scrape the mixture into a bowl and fold in the cheese. Season to taste.

chermoula

2 tsp ground cumin

2 tsp ground coriander

1 tsp smoked sweet paprika

1 tsp cayenne powder

2 garlic cloves, crushed with
1 tsp salt

rind of a preserved lemon,
finely chopped

1 tsp grated ginger root

4 tbsp olive oil

a handful each of flat-leaf parsley
and coriander

This is a North African herb and spice mixture used to marinate and flavour. The measurements here are meant as a guide. Add a tablespoon of water or more to loosen the sauce if you need to.

1 Combine the cumin, coriander, paprika, cayenne, garlic, lemon and ginger in a bowl. Gradually whisk in the olive oil until you have a smooth sauce. Add the parsley and coriander and mix in.

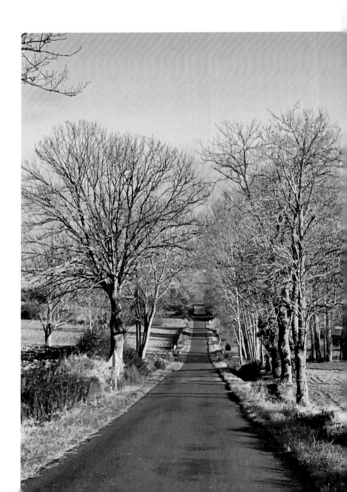

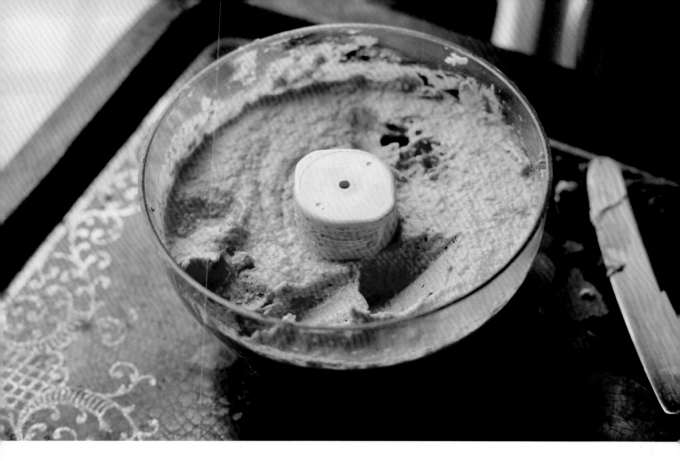

red pepper hummus

SERVES 4

1 red pepper

400g/14oz tin of chickpeas, drained

2 garlic cloves, crushed

3 tbsp tahini

2 tbsp lemon juice

1 tsp smoked paprika, plus an extra
pinch to serve

3 tbsp olive oil

salt and freshly ground black pepper

*A simple variation on this classic dip from the Levant and common to the
countries bordering the eastern Mediterranean, such as Israel, Egypt, Lebanon,
Syria and Greece. The addition of a roasted red pepper changes the colour and
gives it an agreeable smoky edge.*

1 Preheat the oven to 200°C/400°F.

2 Place the pepper on a lightly oiled baking tray lined with foil. Roast
   for about 40 minutes, or until nicely blackened. Slip it into a plastic
   bag and let it cool down. Slide it out of the bag and onto a plate.

3 Now the fun bit – peel the pepper out of its skin, discarding the
   skin as you go. Carefully slice the pepper open and discard the
   seeds. Roughly chop the flesh.

4 Place all the ingredients, except the oil, in a food processor and
   pulse to blitz. With the motor running, slowly pour in the oil, until
   smooth. Season with salt and pepper and transfer the mixture to a
   bowl. Sprinkle with a pinch of paprika to serve.

gremolata

SERVES 2

1 tsp lemon zest

1 garlic clove, very finely chopped

1 tbsp chopped flat-leaf parsley

This is a simple fresh green relish to sprinkle on more or less anything to make it sing.

1 Combine all the ingredients and sprinkle wherever you wish.

a yoghurt sauce

SERVES 4

100g/3½oz Greek yoghurt

100g/3½oz crème fraîche

2 garlic cloves, crushed

2 tbsp lemon juice

3 tbsp olive oil

20g/¾oz flat-leaf parsley

30g/1oz coriander

salt, to taste

Good with most things roasted.

1 Put all the ingredients in a food processor and whizz.

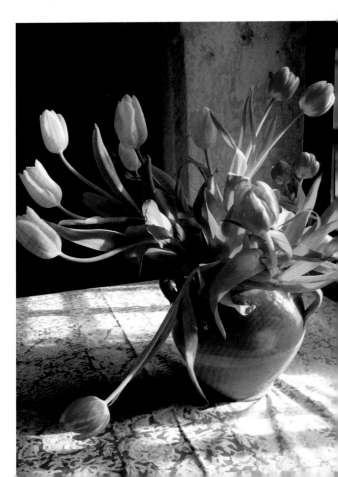

quick all-purpose tomato sauce

SERVES 4

2 tbsp olive oil

2 garlic cloves, thinly sliced

2 sprigs of rosemary

2 x 400g/14oz tins of plum tomatoes, drained and roughly chopped

salt and freshly ground black pepper

A handy everyday sauce. I made this in a jiffy this morning to use 70g of it for the tortino (see p.88). That left plenty for our pasta tonight, giving me time to follow some of today's stage in the Tour de France!

1 Heat the oil in a large pan over a medium heat. Add the garlic and the rosemary and cook for a few seconds, until the garlic starts to sizzle. Add the tomatoes and cook over a medium–high heat, stirring often, for about 15 minutes, until the loose liquid has evaporated and little pockmarks appear on the surface. If you can part the Red Sea – running a spoon through it – it's done.

2 Remove the rosemary sprigs.

3 Season with salt and pepper. *Voilà!*

tomato salsa

SERVES 4

4 large ripe tomatoes, skinned, deseeded and diced

½ red onion, chopped into small dice

1 green chilli, deseeded and chopped into small dice

juice of 1 lime

2 tbsp chopped coriander

salt and freshly ground black pepper

This is a refreshing side salad/sauce with a kick and one that looks beautiful on the plate. Finely chopped fresh and raw ingredients are seasoned with salt and black pepper and finished with lime juice. Try it served with a simple cheese omelette – a flash of colour with the yellow – or as a dip for the chickpea flatbread or a hull-like leaf of endive.

1 Combine all the ingredients in a bowl, season with salt and pepper, and leave the flavours to get to know each other.

tapenade without anchovies

SERVES 6

200g/7oz black olives, pitted

2 tbsp capers

2 garlic cloves, crushed

1 tsp thyme leaves

1 tbsp Dijon mustard

juice of 1 lemon, plus extra if needed

120ml/½ cup olive oil

black pepper

This classic Provençal black-olive dip – cousin to the Green Olive and Artichoke Dip (see p.206) – usually includes anchovies. I've found that it is delicious and useful without them. It's important to use the plumpest, tastiest olives you can find – I think the oily, fleshy Greek ones are best.

1 Put all the ingredients except the oil in a food processor. With the motor running, gradually pour in the oil, bringing the mixture to a nice, nobbly sludge – that is, not too smooth. Taste for balance – you may need a little more lemon juice.

2 Pour the tapenade into a bowl or plastic box and dribble in a little more olive oil to form a preserving film. It keeps in the fridge for a week or more but always bring it back to room temperature before serving.

a simple vinaigrette pour tous les jours

SERVES 4–6

1 tbsp red wine vinegar

juice of ½ lemon

3 tbsp olive oil

salt and freshly ground black pepper

As the title suggests, this is our everyday salad dressing and it's so simple to make.

1 Put a little salt and pepper in a screwtop jar. Add the ingredients, secure the lid and shake to combine.

tomato coulis

SERVES 4

6 tbsp olive oil

6 small shallots, thinly sliced

6 garlic cloves, crushed

2kg/4½lb tomatoes, cored, skinned and roughly chopped

2 sprigs each of thyme and rosemary wrapped in a bay leaf and tied with string

salt and freshly ground black pepper

It's the second week of September and the market stalls are laden with tomatoes. Some are in better shape than others. The less-than-perfect tomatoes are cheap and ripe, and crying out to be coaxed gently into a smooth all-purpose sauce: a coulis.

1 Heat the oil in a large saucepan over a medium-low heat. Add the shallots and garlic and cook for 5 minutes, until softened. Add the tomatoes and the herbs. Turn everything over and bring up to a simmer, then leave to cook, stirring occasionally, until the sauce emerges.

2 It is ready when you can pull your spoon through the mixture to see the bottom of the pan – the parting of the Red Sea. The flavour is concentrating as it cooks.

3 Check the seasoning.

4 When the sauce has cooled completely, remove the herbs; then pour it carefully into a food processor and whizz until smooth.

aubergine and tomato dip with capers and green olives

SERVES 4

1 large aubergine

1 small sweet onion, very finely diced

2 tbsp capers, chopped

12 pitted green olives, chopped

2 garlic cloves, crushed with a pinch of salt

3 large ripe tomatoes, skinned, deseeded and diced small

2 tbsp olive oil

1 tbsp red wine vinegar

pinch of dried oregano

salt and freshly ground black pepper

This smoky aubergine mash with ripe tomato dice can also serve as a handy side salad.

1 If you have a gas hob, place the aubergine on the lowest flame. Turn the aubergine as the skin chars, until it is black all over and the flesh yields easily to the tip of a knife. Leave to cool.

2 If you do not have a gas hob, heat the oven to 200°C/400°F. Place the aubergine on a baking tray and cook until the flesh is soft to the tip of a knife. Leave to cool.

3 When the aubergine is cool, peel it carefully and put the flesh in a mixing bowl. Mash it, then add the remaining ingredients and season with salt and pepper.

spicy moroccan dip

SERVES 4

2 red peppers

1–2 spicy green chillies

8 ripe tomatoes

4 garlic cloves, sliced

4 tbsp olive oil

1 tbsp smoked paprika

1 tsp salt

The Arabic word matbucha *(the Moroccan name for this dip) literally means 'cooked salad'.*

1 Preheat the oven to 200°C/400°F.

2 Place the red peppers and green chillies on a shallow baking tray and put in the middle of the oven. Cook for about 30 minutes, until they have blackened nicely.

3 Take the tray out of the oven and slide the peppers into a plastic bag and seal it. When they have cooled, open the bag and carefully peel off the skin, deseed and roughly chop them. Set aside.

4 Place the tomatoes in a bowl and pour over boiling water. Wait 1 minute and then pour off the water. Peel and chop the tomatoes.

5 Put the tomatoes and garlic in a medium pan and place over a low heat. Cook for 10 minutes to soften. Add the olive oil, chopped peppers and chillies, the paprika and salt.

6 Cook on a low heat for 90 minutes, stirring occasionally as it thickens to stop it burning. Leave to cool and allow the flavours to get to know each other.

green tarator sauce

SERVES 3 OR 4

80g/3oz tahini

15g/½oz flat-leaf parsley

1 garlic clove, crushed

3 tbsp lemon juice

salt

I've read that this loose little sauce from Lebanon traditionally doesn't have garlic in it. I like garlic so I include it, which I've also read is not a capital offence in Beirut. Good with roasted vegetables like the cauliflower recipe on p.37.

1 Put all the ingredients in a food processor. With the motor running, slowly pour in 80ml/⅓ cup of water, whizzing until smooth.

harissa sauce

SERVES 4

1 red pepper

½ tsp coriander seeds

½ tsp cumin seeds

½ tsp caraway seeds

1½ tbsp olive oil, plus extra
if necessary

1 small red onion, roughly chopped

3 garlic cloves, roughly chopped

3 hot red chillies, deseeded and
roughly chopped

1½ tsp tomato paste/purée

2 tbsp lemon juice

½ tsp salt

There are several recipes in the book that call for harissa paste. It is readily available commercially now, but here is a recipe if you fancy having a go at making it yourself.

1 Follow the instructions for cooking, peeling and deseeding the red pepper in the recipe for *Spicy Moroccan Dip* (see opposite).

2 Place a frying pan over a low heat and lightly toast the coriander, cumin and caraway seeds for 2 minutes. Remove them to a mortar and using a pestle, grind to a powder.

3 Heat the olive oil in a frying pan over medium-low heat and fry the onion, garlic and chillies for 10–12 minutes, until the onion and garlic soften and take on some colour.

4 In a food processor, blend all the ingredients together to a sauce, adding more oil as needed.

5 You can keep this in the fridge for a couple of weeks.

lightly spiced nuts

250g/9oz nuts of your choice

1 tsp olive oil

1 tsp salt

several grindings of black pepper

¼ tsp cayenne pepper

Not strictly speaking a sauce or a dip, but a delicious way to roast nuts: use almonds, cashews or hazelnuts.

1 Preheat the oven to 180°C/350°F.

2 Put the nuts in a bowl, add the oil and turn over to coat thoroughly. Add the salt, pepper and cayenne. Mix again.

3 Spread out the mixture on a shallow baking tray. Roast near the top of the oven and test for doneness after about 10 minutes, by picking out a couple from the tray, waiting a minute for them to cool and then testing for crunchiness. If they are still a little soft, return the tray to the oven for another couple of minutes.

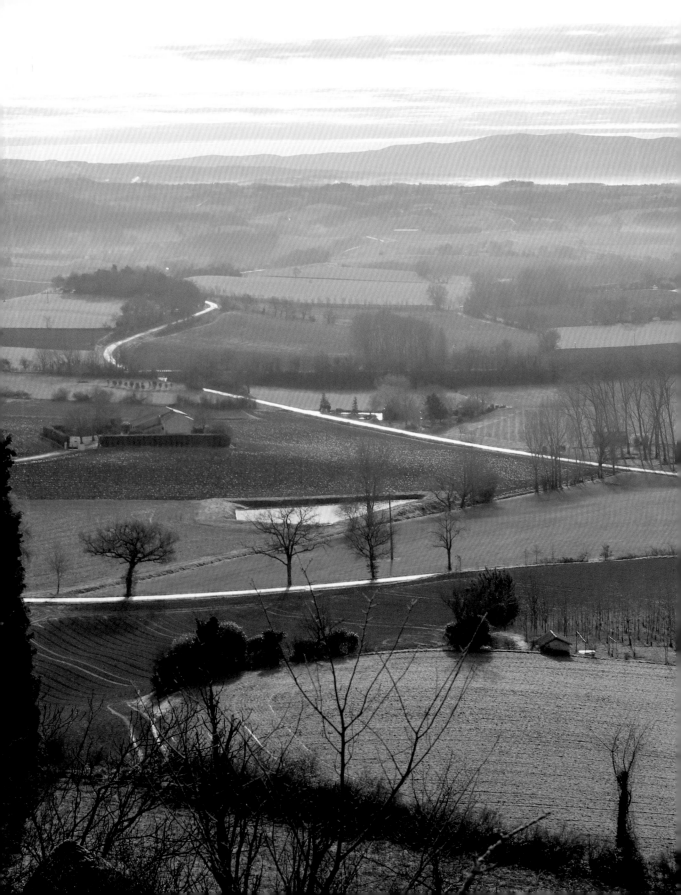

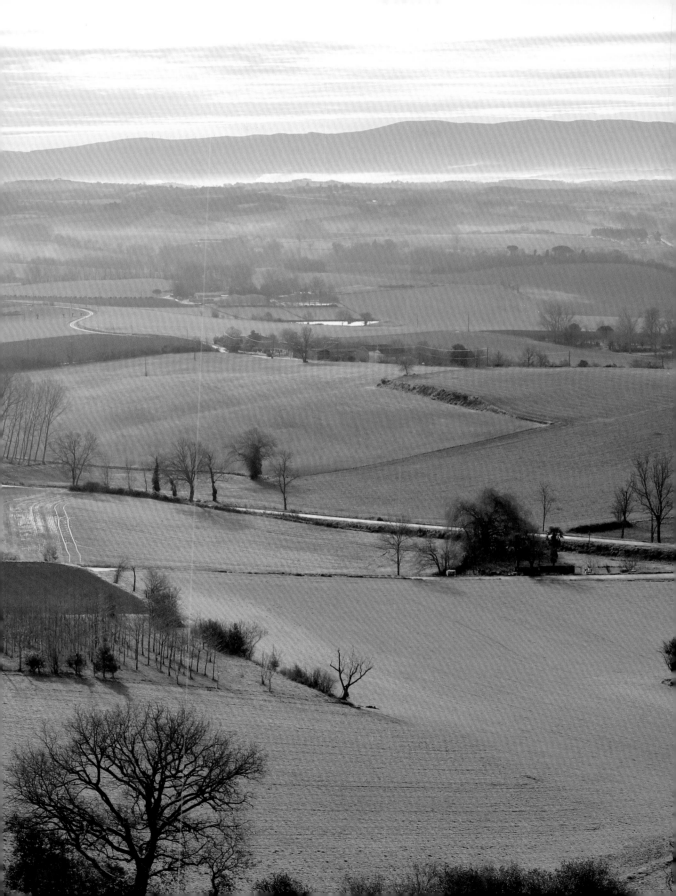

the GI and the GL

The Glycaemic Index (GI) is a measure, on the scale of 1 to 100, ranking carbohydrates according to their effect on our blood glucose levels and thus their post-meal impact.

The Glycaemic Load (GL) is a measure of the impact of the glucose in a single portion of food.

The GI Foundation neatly sums it up thus: 'Not all carbohydrate foods are created equal, in fact they behave quite differently in our bodies. The glycaemic index or GI describes this difference by ranking carbohydrates according to their effect on our blood glucose levels. Choosing low GI carbs – the ones that produce only small fluctuations in our blood glucose and insulin levels – is the secret to long-term health, reducing your risk of heart disease and diabetes and is the key to sustainable weight loss.'

LIQUID CONVERSIONS

IMPERIAL	METRIC	AMERICAN
½ fl oz	15 ml	1 tablespoon
1 fl oz	30 ml	⅛ cup
2 fl oz	60 ml	¼ cup
4 fl oz	120 ml	½ cup
8 fl oz	240 ml	1 cup
16 fl oz	480 ml	1 pint

In British, Australian and often Canadian recipes an imperial pint is 20 fl oz. American recipes use the American pint measurement, which is 16 fl oz.

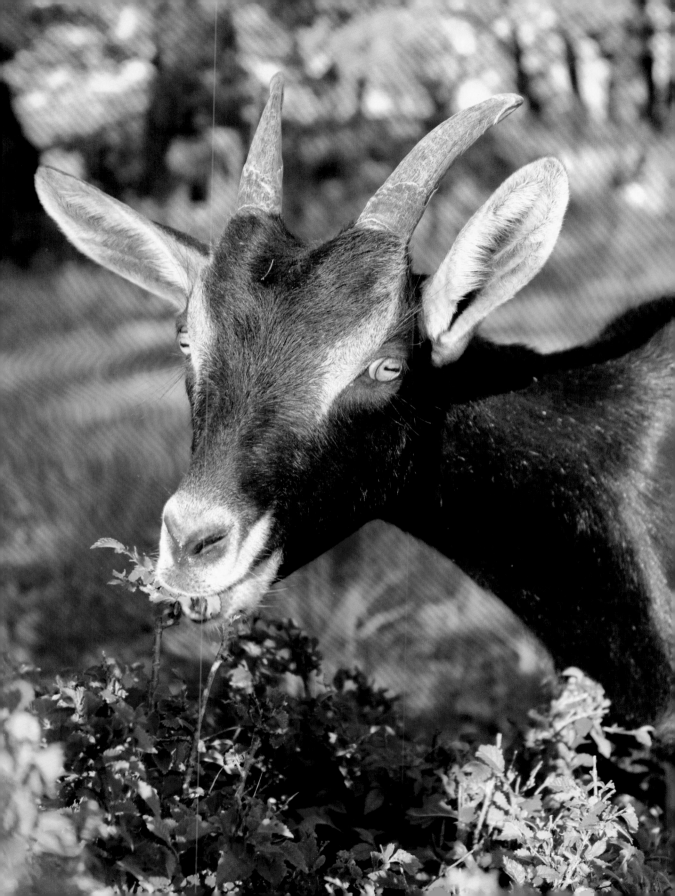

index

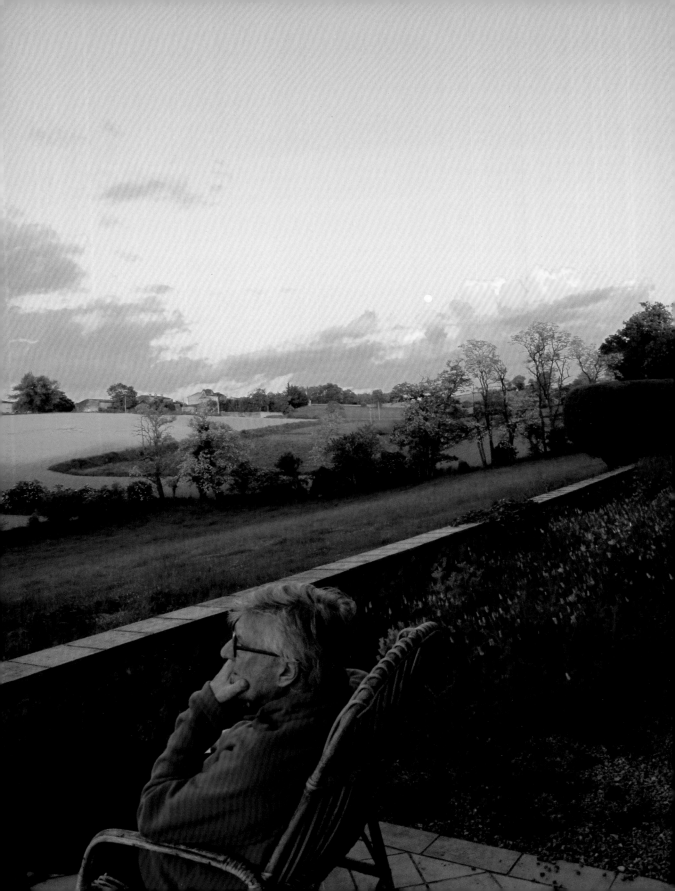